Flexibility

Fastest Scientific Flexibility Program for Middle Splits

(Poses and Practices for Improving Full-body Mobility Over Time)

David Shaw

Published By **John Kembrey**

David Shaw

All Rights Reserved

Flexibility: Fastest Scientific Flexibility Program for Middle Splits (Poses and Practices for Improving Full-body Mobility Over Time)

ISBN   978-1-77485-950-6

No part of this guidebook shall be reproduced in any form without permission in writing from the publisher except in the case of brief quotations embodied in critical articles or reviews.

Legal & Disclaimer

The information contained in this ebook is not designed to replace or take the place of any form of medicine or professional medical advice. The information in this ebook has been provided for educational & entertainment purposes only.

The information contained in this book has been compiled from sources deemed reliable, and it is accurate to the best of the Author's knowledge; however, the Author cannot guarantee its accuracy and validity and cannot be held liable for any errors or omissions. Changes are periodically made to this book. You must consult your doctor or get professional medical advice before using any of the suggested remedies, techniques, or information in this book.

TABLE OF CONTENTS

Chapter 1: The Importance Straching

Stretching isn't just physically based however, it can also be a source of flow into every aspect of your health. It can increase the amount of your body's ability to move, and improve the level of living, and can even impacting your mental well-being. It's what allows your body to perform the exercises that help you attain your fitness goals. It also can serve as an instrument to help you calm your mind in the midst of the ups and downs of life. The best part is that this is only scratching the level of the benefits stretching can bring to your daily routine.

Exercise

The purpose of stretching is to lengthen the muscles. It lets your muscles work more effectively. By stretching, it increases the flexibility of your body which is crucial for exercising. When you exercise, you're working your muscles, which is why they must be in top shape. The ability to move more will improve your exercise since you won't be limited by tight muscles as you'll be able to work many more muscles and improve the quality of your exercise.

Flexibility is not often thought of as a thing that is linked to strength. It's a lie and if you're not convinced me, take a look at the people who practice yoga. Both men as well as women have their bodies toned as well as a substantial level of physical strength. Flexibility isn't the only thing that can be used in the same as strength training, but since muscles collaborate throughout your life, you're better able to make the most of your strength training when you're more flexible.

Stretching isn't a warm-up like we've commonly believed. It is true that you'll see better results by stretching when your muscles have already warm. The best thing to do is to do a five-minute walk or jog through the neighborhood to help your muscles move and then start stretching. Your muscles will feel more relaxed and you'll benefit more from the stretching routine. If you'd like to are able to continue with your other workouts and your muscles will be supple and flexible. If we incorporate stretching into our daily routine nearly guarantees an improvement in the risk of injury when doing any exercise or putting pressure to our muscle. Muscles aren't as likely get tense and can be able to

2

move from one position to another more quickly.

General Living

The lifestyles we lead today are sedentary, which means that we do not move much. Most of us are at our desks the majority of the time. The largest part that is mobile in our bodies is our hands, doing their work on the keyboard. This is not healthy for our muscles. In fact, sitting in the chair for the majority of the day is likely to cause tighter muscles in the hamstrings. This isn't to say that you need to give up your career and turn into an athlete in order to stay healthy however, balance is essential to maintain your body's health.

The balance is achieved by adding stretching to your routine. Sometimes we get distracted by our hectic daily routine that we fail to perform the things that are good for our bodies. If you've ever been suffering from stiff joints, stiffness or pain in particular muscles, even though you're not sure what you did to cause the feeling, you need to be aware that it is the direct result of an inability to move the muscles you use.

Mobility can help you perform your everyday tasks easily. The inability to bend to grab something off the floor or from a low shelf due to stiff muscles isn't the most pleasant feeling. Moreover, it hinders the process of living your life to the fullest. An ideal life is one that has as few constraints as you can. We all want to be able to be able to live our lives as we wish and our bodies shouldn't be the obstacle that keeps us from doing what we want to do. This is exactly why mobility and flexibility are crucial.

As we age our joints and muscles naturally become stiffer. Stretching your muscles to increase flexibility actually slows the process. Start today and you'll make you feel grateful in the near future. Everyone wants to enjoy things we enjoy and don't want age to hinder us from living our lives. The earlier you begin with stretching, the better it'll help you. But don't overlook that stretching can be beneficial out in older age, as stretching can be extremely beneficial for anyone who does it, regardless of the age.

One of the benefits of stretching is stronger and healthier muscles. If our muscles are strong and our posture improves, so does our posture. Slouching is a frequent issue nowadays, and can result in back pain and neck pain. back. In extreme instances, it may result in exhaustion and shortness of breath. If we are able to stretch our muscles, this helps to maintain the correct posture of the muscles which raises our bodies and minimizes the danger of slumping and poor posture.

Another advantage to stretching out is it boosts the flow of blood through our bodies. This means that our muscles will be in a position perform better due to the increased flow of blood towards our muscles. In addition to the increase in blood flow is an increase in nutrients, which means that the supply of nutrients to our muscles will be greater. Additionally, you'll notice less soreness due to the an increase in the amount of blood and nutrients within your body. Your body will be able work better as a whole.

Mental Wellbeing

In the course of our day, our minds are occupied constantly thinking of issues to solve or a situation to attend to. It can be difficult to find the time to sit down with your thoughts and concentrate on your. The inability to unwind your thoughts and concentrate on something that relaxes your mind can have negative effects on your mental health. When you're constantly in motion you have no time to relax and we all require rest in order to be at our best. The rest you take should be physically as well as mental; however, we often neglect the second.

While we exercise, it's a slow and controlled moves. The focus is on what our body is doing and what we feel. This can give your mind an opportunity to unwind from all the thoughts in your head. It's the chance to take an opportunity to relax, de-stress and catch up on your thoughts. Once you're completed, you'll be more prepared to tackle your next round of tasks.

The tension we carry within our muscles. You may notice the muscles that are knotted, specifically in your shoulders and neck. It's a defense technique employed by our bodies when we are overwhelmed or stressed. It could affect how you perform throughout your day. you'll be uneasy and constantly contemplating the stress you're carrying around in your muscles. Stretching is a great solution to this strain but also will help prevent knots in the near future.

Stress and tension can have an adverse effect on our mental health. What happens in our minds eventually take over other areas of our lives. Do not forget how crucial wellbeing of the mind can be to overall wellbeing and happiness. We must be aware of every aspect of our health.

Chapter 2: Do It Right

It is crucial to start with a point, we must be doing things in a proper manner. While you might probably not have the expertise at the start of your journey, but not knowing the correct technique for stretching could cause damage that is not good. It is important to set your expectations from the beginning, so you know what stretching is and what you can do to obtain the best outcomes. This is my goal for you. I want you to achieve the highest results that you can, and this can only be accomplished by taking the proper manner.

The Correct Form

The correct posture refers to the correct performance of each stretch, which will ensure certain that you be able to get the most benefit from your routine of stretching. A lot of stretching exercises target particular muscle groups, which means that when you stretch you'll know exactly which muscle groups you need to be focusing on. Being aware of the area you feel stretched and how you're stretching all over is essential to being able to get a good exercise.

It is common for stretching to cause muscle tension If you experience this, you'll know you're performing something. But it shouldn't cause discomfort. If you experience discomfort, it is an indication that you're performing something incorrectly or have stretched out too much for your muscles at this moment. When you begin to feel pain, stop, think about what caused the pain and make an effort to avoid the pain next time around. The phrase "no pain is no gain" doesn't apply to this scenario. In fact, pushing yourself too far could cause muscle tears and tissue damage.

Be sure to have enough space to stretch. You don't want to be in mid-stretch only to then get interrupted by a piece furniture or a wall. Most of the time you can't alter a stretch to accommodate an area that is smaller, and even if you do at it, you may not be able to benefit from the stretch. Be sure you understand how to perform the stretch prior to trying it. This will allow you to organize your workout better in terms of form and space. Understanding the direction your body is moving can help facilitate easier transitions and an overall better overall experience.

They are held for approximately 30 seconds or longer; this is to ensure that there is tension in your muscles. Insufficient time could not produce the same impact when you take your time. Stretching isn't focused on speed but rather control, so concentrate upon controlling how you move. this will help you become more aware of the manner in which you execute your moves. Do not rush into and out of your stretches; utilize your breathing as a reference in case you are required to. The slowing of your breathing will help you slow your movements and gain more control.

An effective idea is to look at you in your mirror. This will allow you to assess how you appear while performing the stretch and get up on areas where you're going wrong, much more easily. Examine your posture by looking in the mirror particularly when you're doing new or more challenging stretching exercises. When you feel more relaxed, you can remove yourself from the mirror. If you don't have a mirror in your home, consider recording yourself. The same result can be achieved however, you don't need to be restricted to an area with mirrors.

The ability to get your form and technique correct is among the most crucial actions you can take. This will help prevent injuries and ensure you're getting the most benefit from your stretching. This can reduce the frustration because most people feel they're not making progress However, this is only because they're not performing the right stretches. When you are able to do the exercises correctly you'll have half the battle won. It makes the whole experience more enjoyable and worthwhile.

It takes time

Like many other things in life it's all about perseverance and hard work. You will not be able to become flexible after a couple of stretching sessions. It requires time. Consider this: your body hasn't been flexible all of your existence, and now you'll have to get your muscles re-trained. It may take several months to begin to develop your flexibility, but it's worthwhile and the perseverance will result in a positive outcome at the final.

It is recommended to stretch every day. If you are unable to commit to this at all times, try it three to four times per week. If you don't do regularly enough, you may lose the flexibility you've achieved, so consistency is essential. The time you dedicate to stretching every session is contingent on a variety of variables, but the main factor is to establish an idea of what you want to do and stick to it. Ten minutes of stretching each day is more beneficial over two hour of stretching each week. Be aware that we are teaching your muscles to be an a specific manner.

Create a routine and keep it in a place you don't forget. If you set it as a prioritization, you'll be more likely to stick with it and the more you practice it more often, the better for you. It is definitely beneficial to plan your routine of stretching before you start, and you're much more inclined to adhere with an exercise routine when it's laid out. Make a plan for the week ahead, and know what you'll be doing the entire week. That means you only need to start the routine. This will ensure the consistency. It may seem easy and simple However, many people overlook the basic things like scheduling a stretching routine prior to when they begin or making sure they do it for the whole duration.

It may be difficult in the beginning, but the first time you do anything isn't easy, but just keep working hard and don't be discouraged. The outcome you will see in the end are worthy of the effort and time. The most consistent approach always yields the highest benefits.

The Mobility Test and the Flexibility Test

Flexibility and mobility are two things that go hand-in-hand   But   they're   not interchangeable, which is why it's essential to focus on both. A lot of one, and too little of another may cause injuries later on in the future. Bedosky (2018) is a great example of showing us the distinction between flexibility and mobility. Mobility is concerned with joints and their movement range being able to move them with ease implies that you are able to move your joints around their entire range of motion without pain, discomfort or restrictions. Flexibility is the ability to lengthen of muscles. Good flexibility is the ability be able to bend and stretch your muscles without restriction or tightness. Both require work to master however they must be worked on to achieve the greatest outcomes.

We all require a point to begin, and in order to get started from the right spot it is essential to determine what our current level of ability is. Elorreaga (2018) created a mobility test to aid you in determining the level you're at in terms of flexibility and mobility. The test is split into sections according to what area of your body you are focusing on. Before moving forward on your journey, it's recommended to take the test and determine the areas you should focus on the most and what areas that are tight. I'll walk you through each test and can be performed at your home. This isn't meant to substitute any advice offered by a physiotherapist or doctor At time's end, I'm not for you, so when your health professional has provided you with instructions or advice, you should follow that advice. These tests are meant to give you an assessment of your mobility, however they don't diagnose any medical issues.

Our bodies produce different results depending on whether it's heated up as well as when muscles have a cold. Do these tests first while your muscles feel stiff as it will provide you with an understanding of the flexibility and mobility you experience in your daily life. Do it again after your muscles are able to relax or perhaps following a workout, so you can evaluate.

You might be tempted to skip some that you believe you could easily accomplish; however,

I can tell that your flexibility might surprise you by the extent of your limitations It's worth trying every move to determine where your trouble zones are.

Upper Body Mobility

The following exercises are what determines your flexibility and flexibility in the upper body joints as well as muscles.

Shoulder Flexion

This exercise is designed to increase the shoulder's flexibility and mobility. It will display your ability to lift your arms over your head at an upward angle and away from your body.

Instructions for Testing Flexibility:

* Lay down on the floor with your back flat.

* Stand up with arms raised so that they hang over your head.

* Your arms should lie flat on the ground in front of you, and you should not have to extend your back.

* Your arms shouldn't be bent and your ribs must not be flaring excessively.

If you're not able to achieve this, it could mean that you have tight pecs, tight lats, biceps long heads and triceps, rotator cuff or a low thoracic extension. If you are able to do this, then you've got an excellent flexibility in your overhead.

Instructions for the Mobility Test

* Sit back straight and straight to the ceiling.

The same as in the earlier test. extend your arms until they are over your head.

* They should be in contact with the wall, but without an arch in the back or bent arms or a flared rib cage.

If you're not able to perform this test and you were able to pass the previous test, this suggests that you're suffering from poor overhead mobility. It is possible that you have tight or weak rotator cuffs and serratus anterior and lower traps. If you could accomplish this, then you're blessed with great overhead mobility.

Shoulder Extension

These exercises have been designed in order to measure the strength of your shoulder.

Instructions for the Flexibility Test:

Place your hands behind your back, on a box , or any similar flat surfaces.

* Make sure your palms are smooth against the surface.

* Crouch down.

* You must be able to attain at least 45 degrees between your torso and your arm. 90 degrees if you're an athlete or gymnast in the case where it is required.

Your spine shouldn't be rounded.

If you are able to do this, then you are between good and satisfactory shoulders extension versatility. If you have trouble doing this it could be because you have weak pecs, anterior delts or Biceps.

Instructions for Mobility Tests:

* Grab hold of rods or broomsticks with both hands behind. Try it by putting your knuckles in the direction of towards the upward direction (supine grip) as well as with your hands facing downwards (prone grip).

* Draw the rod or stick up and keep you elbows square.

* It is recommended to get a 90-degree angle or greater.

If you're unable to accomplish this, it could be because you be suffering from weak rotator cuffs posterior delts, lats.

External Rotation

This test will determine how well your shoulders turn to the outside.

Test of Flexibility Instructions:

Place your feet on the ground with your arms straight in front of you. It should be an even line that runs starting from your right hand and going until you left.

* Move your elbows upwards at 90 degrees.

Your palms should be towards the ceiling. The hand's back should be straight to the floor.

* Keep your back straight against the floor.

If you can hold your hands' backs and your back flat against the ground simultaneously then you're in excellent external rotation. If not, you might have an internal rotator that is not as tight.

Internal Rotation

This exercise is designed to test the strength of your shoulders move to the right.

Instructions for Testing Flexibility:

* Lay to your side. Then, move your body to the other side, so that the opposite part of the body is lying in the flooring.

The arm of your body should be approximately 70 degrees away from your body, and your fingers pointing towards the sky.

Then, pivot your arm in such a way that your palm begins sliding towards the floor. move as low as you can.

Your wrist should be bent so that your fingers touch the floor.

If you are able to do this, then you've got excellent internal rotation flexibility. If you are having difficulty doing this the reason is that you have an external rotator that is tight or a insufficient posterior capsule.

Instructions for the Mobility Test:

* Lay the palm of your hand flat against the smaller of your back.

The capula (shoulder blade) should be straight It should not be visible.

* Turn your hand to toward your head.

* Move your other hand up over your head to the side, and then turn your back.

Try to grasp fingers with your hands by moving them upwards with the scapula not sticking out.

If you are able to do this the internal rotation mobility is excellent. If not, you might have a weak teres Major and subscapularis as well as serratus anterior or the lower traps.

Wrist and Finger Extension

This technique is aimed at testing the ability to extend your fingers and wrists.

The test for wrist flexibility instructions:

* Stand on your feet, with your hands flat on the floor.
* Make sure your hands are aligned with your shoulders.
* Make sure your hands are in a straight line and move them forward as much as you are able to.
* Your hands of your hands must be kept firmly on the floor at all times.
If you can accomplish this by pushing your arms over 90 °, you've got great wrist flexibility. Should you not be able to do this, then it suggests that you have a tight wrist.
Finger Extension Test Instructions:
* Put your hands together using your fingers and palms together.
* Slowly slide the palms of your hands away from each other.
* Spread your hands as far as you can, with the entire hands touching.
If you are able to do this and achieve an angle of 90 degrees from your back fingers to the back of your hand, then you're in good shape with your finger flexibility. If not, you'll need to improve it.
The wrist and the fingers Flexion

This test measures the extent to which your fingers and wrists move towards the back.

Instructions for the Flexibility Test:

* As you sit down on your knees and place the back of hand on the ground in between the legs.

* Lean to one side. This is the side your arm is located on. For instance, if you use your left arm move it to the right.

• Roll the fingers into a ball, until you're making an elongated fist. The hand that is on the back is still in the floor.

Then slowly move your body back toward the center. Your arms should be straight.

If you are able to return to the center of your body with your wrist perpendicular to the floor If you can, then your fingers and wrist flexion is at a decent level. If not, you'll have to improve it.

Lower Body Mobility

The next exercises and exercises will concentrate on the lower body , and will help you identify any problematic parts in that region.

Internal Hip Rotation

This test will show how your hips move toward the inside. There aren't many scenarios in which you'd do this at a regular basis, but it's a good idea to do it balance the external hip rotations. These are more frequent.

Instructions:

* Begin by putting yourself in a relaxed squat position. Lower yourself the lowest you are able to.

* Lean to the right , then lower the left knee towards the floor.

Your foot shouldn't be lifted off the floor. It is nevertheless normal for it to shift towards the side.

* Place your knee on the ground.

Repeat the process on the other side.

If your knee is able to touch the floor, then you've got an internal hip rotation that is strong.

For those who aren't able to achieve a resting squat, there's another option you can attempt.

Instructions:

• Lay on your stomach while your legs are bent to the point you're at a 90 degree angle.

* Allow your feet to drop onto on the side of your body in a row.

* Your legs must form an a slant of more than 35 degrees.

If you are able to achieve greater than a 35 degree angle the internal hip rotation is acceptable, however it is better to have a 45-degree angle.

If you could not perform both of these movements It could mean the presence of tight glutes or external rotators.

External Hip Rotation and Flexion

This test will determine how well your hips be able to rotate and move outwards.

Instructions:

* Sit straight with your back against the wall.

Stretch your legs straight to the side and place your left leg on you right knee. The left leg should be positioned to touch the right knee.

* Raise your right knee to the highest you can reach.

* You can repeat the exercise the opposite side in the event you want and see what happens.

If you can bring the right leg (in this instance) close to the chest area, you've got excellent flexibility. But, 45 degrees towards your chest would be sufficient. If you're unable to achieve this it is likely that you have overly tight TFL (tensor fascia lata; a portion of the hip muscles) the piriformis muscle, or glutes.

The Hip Abduction and the External Hip Rotation

This test will determine the extent to which your leg can get away from the midline. You can think of doing a side-kick , or leg lift.

Instructions:

Begin by sitting on the ground on your sit bones. Your rear should lie straight. Make sure you're not sitting on your tailbone.

* Place your feet together to ensure that your feet are in contact.

* Bring your feet towards your body, then try to press your knees until your knees reach the floor.

If you have your feet pulled to the extent that they are able to be, and you are able to bring your knees close to the ground, then you're quite flexible. If not, there is a possibility that you have tight adductors as well as internal rotators.

Hip Extension

A well-extended hip allows your leg to follow ahead of you.

Instructions:

* Place your body on your back on the floor or on a flat surface. The most suitable place is an ottoman or table.

* Your entire back should be exposed with your butt half-on and the other half off.

Your right knee should be brought towards your chest. pull it as close to you can, then push it back to the ground.

* Let you left leg space to hang from the edge. You should bend your knee at about a 90 degree angle.

* Your leg should extend beyond your body's edge at an angle of more than 180 degrees. Your back shouldn't ever be able to leave the surface.

If your leg is hanging over the surface but isn't being pulled upwards, then you're in good shape with your hip extension. If you're not able to extend your hip, it is likely that you suffer from tight hip muscles, or tight quads. If you find that your leg is moving towards the outside, then you have weak adductors, or tight TFL.

Pike

The pike position is essentially the forward bend of your leg, but you will feel it through the muscle of the leg.

Instructions for the Pike Flexibility Test:

* Begin by standing straight and putting your feet together.

* Bend at your hips and keep the back straight.

* Keep your knees locked.

* Try to go down as low as you can while keeping your back straight.

If you are able to get your back to lie at 90 degrees to the legs you've got sufficient pike flexibility. For those who are more flexible you can attempt to bring your palms with the ground approximately two feet away distance from the floor. If you're not able to attain at least 90 degrees angle, it means that you are suffering from tight calves, hamstrings, and Achilles tendon.

Pike Mobility Test Instructions:

* Begin by standing straight.

* You can kick either of your legs to the side without bending your knees as well as your spine.

* Try to get your leg at 90 degrees. Then, stand out in the front of you.

If you're unable to raise your leg to 90 degrees, it is possible that you be suffering from weak hip flexors as well as a weak rectus muscle.

Ankle Dorsiflexion

The movement tests the flexibility that your ankle has. It is crucial to have strong ankles since they are a part of the structure that holds us up and aids in keeping us moving.

Instructions:

Begin by putting yourself into a lunge pose against the wall. Your knee and the toe of one leg must be in contact with the wall while your other leg is in front of you.

* Place a ruler underneath your foot or right beside it.

Step your foot backwards one inch at a time. Your knee should be fixated to the wall.

If you reach 5 inches in height, you can stop. Be sure that the heels of your feet is not lifted above the level of the earth.

If you are able to reach five inches from the wall, that indicates the dorsiflexion of your body is in good shape. If not, it indicates that you might have an Achilles tendon.

If you're experiencing a flexibility or mobility issue with a muscle that you didn't even realize existed, you don't have to be concerned. As long as you are aware the muscle is located in your back , hip or anywhere else, that's acceptable. I'll offer you stretches that take care of all the areas that will surely target the muscle that you've never known about and help improve the problematic region.

Final Thoughts on The Mobility Test and Flexibility Test

After you've completed the test for flexibility and mobility and completed the mobility and flexibility test, you should be able to determine the areas where you have issues. It may seem like a lotof work, however, I'm sure this won't take too time and give you a great assessment of where you are currently. Don't be down if you're unable to perform some or all of these moves and that's why I created this book. I'm here to assist you in your quest of recovering your flexibility and mobility.

To move forward it was necessary to understand what you're doing right now. Once you're aware of the things you're skilled at and what you can make improvements on, we'll begin to provide you with the tools needed to achieve your goals of greater flexibility and mobility.

2

Chapter 3: Conditioning: All The Stretches You Will Ever Need To Know

The exercises discussed throughout this article will concentrate on solving short-term issues. Sometimes we lie down or even sleep in a way that is uncomfortable, which causes joints and muscles to be injured. You're probably waking up with stiff neck after lying in a position that was uncomfortable. This type of situation is quite common and isn't typically a cause of lasting damage, but it can be uncomfortable. If you're in pain or feel sore, it means you'll not be optimally. Stretching is the best method to relieve the discomfort and pain so that you can return to feeling and performing at your best.

The exercises below are broken down into specific body parts stretching exercises for specific body parts. This helps you get through the chapter more easily and, should you experience particular issues then you'll are aware of the answer. Let's move on to the stretching.

Shoulder, Neck and chest

Many suffer from an underlying pain or tightness in these regions. It's usually because of our posture at our computer or sleep.

Whatever the reason it is difficult to manage. The following exercises will assist in relieving stiffness, tension and pain from the neck, chest, and shoulders.

Thread the needle

This stretch is designed to target your shoulder girdle muscles as well as an abdominal muscle known as the pectoralis minor.

Instructions:

Start by kneeling on your feet. Your hands should be in alignment with your shoulders, as well as your knees should be in line with your hips.

* Grab the right hand and extend it out through that space in between the left and thigh. Your palm should point towards the upward direction.

* Relax your left arm to let the right side of your body to experience greater flexibility. You will feel it in the back of your right shoulder.

* Hold for a few seconds, then repeat it a few times more before moving to the opposite side.

Upper Trapezius Stretch

This stretch targets your neck muscles. It provides the muscles with a long stretch.

Instructions:

Begin by sitting down or standing up with your spine straight.

Put one hand on your back. It could be either on your lower back, or in between shoulders.

* Grab another hand, then place it on one side opposite to your head. draw your head toward your shoulder.

* There should be a feeling of tension in your neck, on the opposite side of your arm. and then pull your head back. Do this for 20 to 30 minutes and then repeat it with the opposite arm.

Quruped Thoracic Spinal Stretch

This stretch is targeted at the upper portion of your spine.

Instructions:

Start with all-fours. Place your hands in alignment with your shoulders , and your knees and hips. Your core must be engaged and your back must be straight throughout the day.

* Rub your head's back using your right hand. don't put pressure on your head.

Slowly bring your shoulders and head towards the inside toward your opposite arm.

* Move all the way backwards, over the point of beginning until your elbow is pointed toward the ceiling.

Revert to middle after maintaining it for several seconds.

* Repeat for around 30 seconds, then repeat it with the other side.

Child's Pose

It is a very simple yoga exercise that can help your back, neck, and shoulders. It should also be felt in your hips and glutes.

Instructions:

* Kneel on the ground and then sit down upon your feet. The knees of your feet should slightly larger than your hips as well as your heels should be in contact with each other.

You can fold your body so that your torso will be resting on your legs. Arms out towards the side so that they're above your head. Your forehead should be on the floor.

* Bring your shoulders and chest toward the floor. This can cause a greater stretch.

* Maintain that position for 30 second prior to repeating.

T-spine Windmill Stretch

This stretch targets a variety of muscles of your shoulder.

Instructions:

* Sit on your side , with your arms extended towards the front with your hips and knees bent at 90 degrees.

Place your arms over one another and do the same by crossing your legs.

* Move your upper hand towards the opposite part of the body. you'll now lay with both arms spread out across the opposite side to form an X shape.

* Slowly return back to the beginning position.

Repeat 5-10 times before repeating the opposite side.

Reverse Shoulder Stretch

This workout will focus on your pecs as well as your deltoids.

Instructions:

Begin by putting both of your palms behind, with your palms facing upwards.

* Your arms and back should be straight while you are pulling the shoulder blades towards each other.

• Push your arms up until you feel the tension in your pec muscles.

* Stay in this position for approximately 30 seconds.

Cervical Side Bend

This stretch can help ease tension in neck muscles.

Instructions:

Sit or Stand while keeping your neck and back straight.

* Make sure your right ear is on your right shoulder as you continue to look directly in front of you.

* You will feel the stretching in your left neck muscles. Keep it for a few seconds and then repeat the process on the opposite side.

Cervical Rotation

This stretch is also focused on neck muscles.

Instructions:

Your head should be turned to the side and make sure that you do not shift your shoulders.

* Keep it for a few seconds before turning to the other side.

* If you'd like to increase the pressure, apply pressure with your hands and press against your cheek gently.

Wall Chest Stretch

This allows you to stretch those chest muscles.

Instructions:

* Put an arm straight against a wall.

* Step forward , keeping your leg the farthest from the wall.

Move your chest gently toward the side and feel the stretch in your chest.

* You can move your hands lower or up higher on the wall to spread out the different sections of your chest.

Repeat the process on the opposite side.

Anterior Scalene Stretch

Sometimes neck stiffness can be due to the anterior muscle This stretch will target this muscle.

Instructions:

* Put your right hand over your head.

Begin slowly pulling your head towards the side to ensure that your right ear is closer to your shoulder.

* Keep this posture for 30 seconds, then repeat it three times before moving to the opposite side.

Arms, Hands and Wrists

When stretching we tend to neglect our hands, wrists, and arms. They are nevertheless important areas of our bodies and should not be overlooked. If you're one who works at a computer throughout the day, experiencing any kind of stiffness or discomfort in these areas can hinder your productivity. There are a few exercises which can help ease the pain and aid in getting the mobility you need.

Wrist Extensor Stretch

It is a very popular stretch to ease tension on your wrists.

Instructions:

* Extend your hand towards the side and move your wrist downwards so your palm is in front of you.

* Use the other hand to move your bent wrist towards you with a gentle pull. You will feel the tension in your forearm and wrist.

* For 30 seconds, hold the position and do it three more times. Repeat the process on the other side.

Wrist Flexor Stretch

This stretch is opposite to the stretch you did before. It is a stretch of the muscles that are located on the inside of your arm and wrist.

Instructions:

* Extend your hand to the side with your palm down.

* Bend your wrist upwards.

* Grab the other hand and gently pull your wrist towards yourself until the stretching feels on your forearm.

* For 30 seconds, hold the position and do it three more times. Repeat the process on the other side.

Squeeze Tennis Ball

The stretch is designed to strengthen the muscles and joints in the wrist and hand.

Instructions:

* Take a tennis ball with the palm of your hand, and press it down as intensely as you are able to.

* Keep this position for approximately 4 or 5 seconds , then gradually release.

Repeat this 15 times before switching to the opposite hand

Desk Press

The stretch is targeted at your wrists as well as forearms.

Instructions:

* Locate an office or table where you can put your hands on it with your wrists in a tuck,

making sure that your fingers are pointed towards you.

Push gently to the side until you are able to feel the stretching in your forearm.

* Keep the position for 15 seconds and repeat this 10 times.

Eagle Arms

This stretch is great to stretch your shoulders and wrists.

Instructions:

* Sit or stand straight with your arms straight in the direction of your body.

* Make sure you cross your right and left arms, placing the right hand over the left.

* Turn both elbows to bend them toward the ceiling.

* Twist your arms to ensure that each hand are touching.

Take both arms away from your body with an upward motion and you will feel a swell of your shoulder blades.

* Hold this posture for five deep breaths then change hands.

Assisted Side Bend

This exercise stretches your arms, but it also increases the length of your torso.

Instructions:

* Sit back straight.

* Bend your arms to the point that they are over your head.

* Hold the wrist of one hand and the other hand and bring yourself to the side.

If you feel your ribs tense, move them backwards so that the stretch only feels through your arm and side.

* Keep this position up to 30 secs or so until you feel comfortable and then switch to the opposite side.

Torso and Back

A tight back could limit the range of motion you can experience. These stretches can help you to restore the flexibility of your back.

The Cobra

The stretch will lengthen your upper body, and is perfect for those who suffer from pain that is caused by sitting in a chair for too long.

Instructions:

* Lay on your stomach on the floor.

* Place your hands right beneath your shoulders, breathe into your chest and lift up your hands.

When your arms are straight, you can look to the ceiling and stretch your neck. Do this for around 30 seconds.

Inhale slowly, then exhale, and return to your normal state.

* Repeat this three times.

Hip Hinge

This stretch is especially beneficial for lower back pain.

Instructions:

* Get up, standing straight with both your legs spaced. You should be just a few feet of the wall.

* Keep your hands hanging either to your side or towards the front. Bend your knees slightly and then bend your pelvis, so that your entire body is positioned toward the ground.

* When your back is straight to the ground, slowly lift yourself back to the starting point.

Sphinx Pose

This is a common pose in yoga, and it is utilized in order to build the strength of the spine and stretch the abdomen.

Instructions:

Begin by lying on your back and the uppers of your feet should be facing downwards.

* Pull your arms back and raise yourself so that your shoulders and elbows are aligned. Your palms should rest level with the ground and your forearms must be in a straight line.

* Inhale and then push downwards on your forearms, then raise your chest and head toward the ceiling.

Engage your core and glutes. Push your pelvis to the floor.

* Keep this posture for 10 breaths, then let yourself relax and then bring yourself to a seated position slowly.

Knee-to-chest stretch

This stretch targets the lower back.

Instructions:

* Lay on your back flat and then bring your right knee to your chest.

* Using both hands, grasp the shin of your left leg, and then pull it back to drive this leg directly into your chest. If it's too difficult then extend to your left foot.

Do not raise your hips. Really extend your spine.

* Hold the pose for 5 to 30 minutes Release and repeat it at minimum three times , before moving onto the next leg.

Piriformis stretch

This stretch can help relieve all tension from your back and buttocks and hips.

Instructions:

* Sit on your back, and keep the knees bent.

* Grab your right ankle, and then place it on you left leg.

* Take your left leg and pull it toward your chest. Try to get as close to your chest as you can.

* Hold this position for 30-60 seconds. Repeat the opposite leg.

Pelvic tilt

This stretch will ease stiffness and pain within your back. It can also help strengthen your abdominal muscles.

Instructions:

* Lie on your back on the floor with your knees are bent. The hands must be at your side , with your their palms flat on the floor.

• Flatten your back until it is on the floor and work those core muscles.

* Tent for 5-10 seconds, then release slowly. Repeat at least 5 times. Repeat as many times as you want.

Cat-cow stretch

This exercise stretches your spine as well as your upper body.

Instructions:

* Begin at the bottom of your feet.

Breathe into your chest, push your belly toward the ground, then lift your head.

* Now in one easy motion exhale, pull your chin into the crease and raise your spine towards the ceiling.

Repeat this process for around 60 minutes.

Partial Crunch

This technique can help strengthen your spine if you suffer from back discomfort.

Instructions:

* Lay on your back on your knees bent and your feet placed on your floor.

* Pull your lower body back into the floor, and then engage your core.

* Lift your shoulders and head just a little off the ground, lifting your feet up with your hands. Utilize your muscles in your core and not your neck to help support this move.

* Do this for anywhere from 1 to 3 minutes. Relax, and repeat.

Hips and Glutes

Hips that are tight are something that many struggle with. at times, you'll notice it while sitting. Your glutes are by far the most significant muscle within your body, which is why it is crucial to be aware of it Both these muscles are connected for flexibility and mobility.

The Half-Lord of the Fishes

This stretch is targeted at your spine and hips.

Instructions:

Begin by sitting on the ground, then place your left foot on the right side of your thigh. Then bend your right leg until your foot is closely to your butts as you could reach it.

Your right elbow should be placed to one side of the knee, and put your left hand behind your body to provide support.

* Hold your left foot securely on the ground while you extend.

* Keep the position for minimum 30 seconds, then repeat the same exercise on the opposite side.

Glute Bridge

This exercise stimulates the glutes, and is done via an extension of the hip.

Instructions:

Place your body on your back while keeping your knees bent. your feet spaced hip-width apart.

* Move your pelvis toward the ceiling by energizing your glutes, then drive your heels towards the ground.

* Keep your hand up for 5-10 seconds, and then slowly lower yourself back to the ground. Repeat 10 to 15 times.

Pigeon Pose

This is a great stretch for those who are on their feet often because it can stretch the hips, glutes and the piriformis.

Instructions:

* Begin by getting to your knees on the right side. Bring your left knee down to the left side and then move your right leg in front of you.

* Put your hips on the ground and then move your hands on the ground as long as you are able to. The palms should be facing towards the ground.

* Keep your hips in a straight line.

* Hold this posture for 20-30 seconds. Repeat with the other side.

Stretching in Figure 4 Lie

This movement provides a fantastic stretch to your glutes as well as hip flexors.

Instructions:

* Lay on your back, with your legs bent, and feet above the ground.

• Place the right ankle on the left side of your thigh.

* Hold your left thigh in your hands and pull both legs towards your chest.

* Hold the position for at minimum 20 minutes. Repeat on the opposite side.

Sungine with Spinal Twist

This exercise will stretch the hip flexors and back muscles and quads

Instructions:

* Stand straight with your feet in a straight line, then take a huge step forward using your right leg.

* Drop your right knee until you're in a squat position. Back leg must be extended to the side.

* Place your hand to the left on the ground for security and reach for the ceiling using your right hand. This will result in your back to turn. Pay attention to with your left hand.

* Hold for at minimum 30 minutes. Repeat on the left side.

90/90 Stretch

This stretch is intended to release the tightness in the hips.

Instructions:

* Sit down on the floor, with your left leg extended towards the front and bend it to 90 degrees. It should lie straight on the ground with your foot bent and in the direction of your right.

The right side of your knee should move to the left as you bend your knee. extend your foot. It should point to the side.

* Your left cheek should be touching the ground. Now, attempt to bring your right cheek as near to ground as it is possible by bending your hips downwards.

* Stay for at minimum 30 seconds before repeating for the opposite side.

Lunging Hip Flexor Stretch

This stretch can open up the hips.

Instructions:

* Sit down to one knee. One leg should be placed facing you at 90 degrees, and the other bent behind you with the feet's tops laid flat on the ground.

* Try to lean forward to push your hips toward the floor.

* squeeze your butt and raise your arm to the opposite side of your leg.

* For 30 seconds, hold the position for 30 seconds, and then repeat the exercise on the opposite side.

Thighs and Knees

Knee pain can get into the way of our daily life. If you feel tension in our thighs, this could cause discomfort in knees. These exercises can aid in relieving pain in your knees and thigh area.

Quad Stretch

The purpose of this stretch is to relieve muscle tension within the quads which may be felt around the knee region.

Instructions:

* Lay on your back with your legs placed over each other. Make use of the arm closest to the ground to help you stand up.

* Bend your leg to the knee, then grasp your foot with your hands.

* Move your foot towards your back until you can feel the quad muscles stretch.

* Keep this position for at most 30 seconds and repeat it on the opposite side.

Side Lunge

This stretch will target the adductors (inner thigh muscles).

Instructions:

* Begin to get in the lunge side by stretching one leg to the side , and then bend the knee to the side.

* Make sure to keep the entire foot of the leg that is stretched on the floor as possible.

* You can put your fingers on the ground in case you require extra stability.

* Try to get to the lowest level you possibly can and hold it for 15 to 30 seconds, then repeat the opposite side.

Supine Hamstring Stretch

This stretch is great for your hamstrings within your thighs.

Instructions:

* Sit on your back and keep you knees bent.

• Use the towel or resistance bands to wrap around your thigh, and push it towards your. The other leg may be bent or straighten it to get greater stretch.

Try to maintain the leg you pull as straight as you can.

* Keep the body in as tight a position as you can in 30 to 60 minutes. Repeat 3 times, and then move to the opposite side.

Wide-Legged Forward Fold

This stretch targets the muscles in your thighs.

Instructions:

* Keep your legs between 3 and 4 feet apart. It may be wider or shorter in accordance with your height.

Straighten up and put your feet down on the ground. Your feet should be parallel , not facing towards the inside.

* Breathe in and, when you exhale you can bend your hips, while keeping your back straight and straight.

* Reach towards the ground with your fingers, making sure you get yourself as near to the ground as you can.

* Keep in this posture for at most five minutes.

The Knight Stretch

The purpose of this stretch is to stretch your thighs and widen your hips.

Instructions:

* Take a step into the lunge posture, with one leg bent downwards behind you, and the other bent to the front.

Breathe in, pull your chest forward, then move your hips forward. Then stretch it to the maximum extent you can.

* Keep it for 30 seconds, then repeat five times per side.

Lower leg, Ankles as well as Feet

These areas of our bodies constitute the foundation of your body and must be sturdy. Intense ankles can result in pain while walking, which is why it's vital to regain mobility in these parts of the body.

Tip Toe Tense

This stretch will cover to the entire lower leg region.

Instructions:

• Stand up straight, then step up onto your toes.

* Hold the position for 5 seconds, then slowly bring yourself back in a controlled and slow manner.

* Repeat this process about 10-15 times.

Ankle Rotation

This technique can ease ankle stiffness.

Instructions:

* You could be lying down or sitting during this maneuver.

Get your heel off the floor and then rotate you ankle left to right. keep it for a few seconds.

* Now, turn your ankle to the left and hold it for several minutes.

* You can repeat this repeatedly as often as you want. Repeat on the opposite foot.

Ankle pull (Band Stretch)

This stretch can help to loosen the ankle.

Instructions:

* Sit on the ground and straighten your legs to the side.

* Grab a small towel or resistance, and wrap it on your foot.
* Pull on the band, pulling your foot towards your.
* Keep your foot in place for 10 seconds before releasing and repeat the 10 up to 15 times. Repeat on the opposite foot.

Toe Grip Challenges

This workout will strengthen the muscles in your toes and feet.

Instructions:

* You could use things like a towel or even a small piece of object such as marbles for help with this.
* Lay your object onto the ground and try to hold it with your toes.

Repeat this gripping motion at least 10 times before repeating with the opposite foot.

Chapter 4: Massage Bolls And Foam Rollers

We're all sure to have had some kind of tightness in our muscles which make us uncomfortable and stiff. This isn't comfortable, and we'd like to rid ourselves of it as fast as we can to regain the fully-range of motion. There are several tools we can utilize to help us with this. The foam roller and the massage ball are specifically designed to relieve knots and stiffness from our muscles.

The connective tissue of your body that joins the bones, muscles and ligaments is known as fascia. When they tighten, it is the reason for the stiffness that you may be experiencing. In this situation knots and trigger points create that cause pain. the most effective way to relieve the trigger points is by massaging them away and this is known as self-myofascial release. Here is where foam roller and the massage ball are available. If you're not looking to spend money on an massage ball or foam roller, a tennis ball can be just as effective.

Locate the part which has knots or a painful area. After that, grab your foam roller or ball. You'll need to lay on the object, or place it on the wall and gently move it around over the knot. The force will allow it to be massaged. Foam rollers are ideal for larger areas and balls target particular regions. Regularly using them will help prevent injuries and discomfort that could arise in the future. It's also a good method of lengthening and warming muscles prior to stretching.

If you've got the funds to invest some more money on something that is going to benefit you by massages and removing knots, then I'd suggest getting a TheraGun. It utilizes a combination of vibrations and force to alleviate stiffness and pain as well as expand the flexibility. It accomplishes all of this without needing to do anything close to the same amount of effort as you would with foam rollers, massage balls.

3

Repetition: Stretching Routines that Let You Recover More Fast

M

Most of us will suffer at the least some minor muscle injuries or sprains throughout our lives. These may be due to fitness, lifestyle and flexibility issues or from an health issue. It's almost unavoidable, however there are some specific practices to help us get over the challenges faster, meaning we don't get trapped in this place for long.

Procedures to prevent injuries, sprains as well as aches and discomforts

Minor injuries and sprains even though they're not considered to be severe, could cause issues and cause us to slow down significantly. Let's look at some of the routines that could assist us in recovering from these injuries more quickly.

Calf Routine

This is a very common injury that happens when you apply too much pressure on your calf muscle , or overexert it. Look over the steps below to assist. It's not necessary to do everything simultaneously, which could cause too much stress on your muscles. Instead, start with the initial few , and gradually add to your workouts as you become stronger.

Calf Stretch 1:

* Sit on the floor with your legs extended to the side.

* Put a towel or a roll of an up-rolled towel under your ankle to raise it.

* Take an elastic belt or strap and then place it on your upper foot, right below your toes.

* Pull this strap until the band is stretched. You may feel a some discomfort but not excessively.

* Keep it for 30 seconds, then repeat 3 times.

Calf Stretch 2:

* Take a band of resistance Choose the one with the lowest resistance and put it on your foot. The towel or roll remains under your ankle.

* Press your toes up in the direction of the resistance band.

Then gradually raise your foot using controlled movements.

* Repeat 10 times in the beginning. If you can, raise your reps to around 15 or 20.

Calf Stretch 3:

* Lay on your back and bend your bottom leg forward and raise your upper leg from the floor.

You can stretch your foot and you will notice it in the calves. Then, point your toe slightly towards the floor.

• Lift your leg and down again in one move It's not necessary to raise it high.

* Lower your leg to the ground in one smooth movement.

Start with between 10 and 15 and gradually increase the number if it's easy for you. You can add weights if you require additional support.

Calf Stretch 4:

* Sit down in a chair and hold it to the back.

* Step back with one leg , so that it's spread out behind you. Another leg must be bent slightly towards the front. Toes pointed inward.

* Lean forward into the front of your leg. Keep it for 30 seconds, then repeat the exercise three times.

Calf Stretch 5:

* Start in the exact position as in the previous exercise, however instead of being straight in the back bent slightly, bend it a bit.

Lean back and stretch the muscles. The stretch is targeted at the soleus muscle, which is located below the calf. This is the place you'll feel it.

* Keep it for 30 seconds, then repeat 3 times.

Calf Stretch 6:

Follow the steps on this Tip Toe Tense stretch mentioned in the previous chapter.

* Begin with around 10 repetitions. Increase it when you feel that you are able.

The next exercises are slightly more challenging, but only perform these at the conclusion of your recovery if you feel that your muscles have sturdily to a certain extent.

Calf Stretch 7:

* Sit in a squat position, then lower yourself into the squat position.

* Once you've brought your body back, you can extend the motion until you are on your feet.

* All of this should be a fluid, controlled motion.

Start by doing five, and gradually begin to work your way up.

Calf Stretch 8:

* Squat into the lunge position, one foot in front, the one behind.

* Stand on your toes and stand on both feet.

* Bend your knee back to the side, then raise yourself back up.

* This should be done in one fluid movement.

Begin with five then, as you get at ease increasing the number you're doing.

Hamstring Routine

Hamstrings are an ordinary muscle that can become quite tight and may be injured or pulled during exercises. If you suffer from a injury to your hamstrings, then this routine can help you get back to full strength.

Hamstring Stretch 1:
* Lay on your stomach and support your body using your elbows.
* One of your feet should be lifted as high as you are able to lower the other in one smooth movement.
* Start with ten and then see if you can grow it from there.
Hamstring Stretch 2:
Keep your belly on and raise your foot until it is pointing toward your butt.
Keep the movement gradual and controlled.
Start with ten, then increase it if you believe you are able to do more.
Hamstring Stretch 3:
* Roll onto your back, then bend your knees.
* Take your hips off the ground , and slowly lower it back down.
Start with ten begin to work your way up.
* Try to make it more difficult by finishing the single-leg version
Hamstring Stretch 4:
* Step into the lunge position and then begin to perform a simple lunge.

* Lift your body down and up in one smooth motion Do this slowly.

* Do ten times and begin to work up in the event that you are able to.

Quad Routine

The quads are usually strained when the force of a lot is put on them, usually due to inflexibility or sports. If you've got an injured quad, follow the following exercise a few times throughout the day until the quad heals.

Quad Stretch 1:

• Lay on your stomach and grasp your ankle or use a belt secure your ankle while you pull it towards your butt.

* Pull as hard as you can. Hold at least 30 seconds. Repeat this three times.

Quad Stretch 2:

* Sit on your knees and put your foot in front bent at a 90-degree angle.

* Take your back foot, and then bring it to your butt, if prefer a greater stretch in your foreleg.

* Stay for 30 seconds, then repeat three times.

Quad Stretch 3:

* Stand up and keep the back straight.

Bend your foot in such a way that it is moving towards your butt. Grab the foot with your hands and push it down into your butt.

* Ensure that both of your knees are aligned.

* Stay for 30 seconds, then repeat 3 times.

Glute Strain

The strain on your glutes can result because of sitting too long or from exercising in a strange way. If you are experiencing muscle strain in your glutes you should follow this workout.

Glute Stretch 1:

• Lay down on your back, with your knees bent. Take a hold your thigh under your body and pull it toward your body.

* You will feel the stretching in your glutes.

* Keep it the position for 30 second, then repeat three times each on the opposite side.

Glute Stretch 2:

Follow the steps for the Lying Stretch shown in Figure 4 in the previous chapter.

* If you'd like to get more stretch out Instead of lying flat, you can do it standing up.

* Use your hands to support behind you , and then use the leg that is on the ground to bring the bent leg closer to your chest.

* Keep it until you are able to hold for 30 seconds. then repeat three times each on the opposite side.

Glute Stretch 3:

* Lay on your stomach, and squeeze your butt tight.

* Lift your leg back.

* Keep it for 3 seconds, then relax, then repeat ten times.

Groin Strains

A groin strain can be an injury to the muscles of your adductor in your legs. They are located in the inner thigh. If you suffer from an injury to your groin. Follow the following exercises.

Groin Stretch 1.

* Sit on the floor, and bring your feet in a way that your feet's soles are in contact.

* Grab your elbows and press down on your inner thighs.

* Lean forward toward your feet.

* Stay for 30 seconds, then repeat three times.

* If you'd like to stretch your thigh move your feet towards you.

Groin Stretch 2.

* Sit down on one knee and place the other leg straight in front of you.

* Move the leg towards the side so far as is comfortable for you.

* Push forward using your hips.

* Keep your hand in place for 30 seconds, then repeat three times for each leg.

Groin Stretch 3.

Straighten up and move your feet toward the front and outward at an angle of 45 degrees.

You should push yourself up to the front of your leg.

* Keep it for 30 seconds, then repeat three times.

Shoulder Pain

If we place too excessive weight on our shoulders, or rest on our shoulders this can result in shoulder discomfort. If you are suffering with shoulder discomfort, you should follow this procedure.

One Shoulder Stretch:

* Bend and then grasp a chair and let your arms hang to the side.

You can swing your body like a pendulum. Your entire body should be moving not only your arm.

* If you would like your shoulder to stretch slightly, put an object in your hand.

* Repeat this for a couple of minutes.

Shoulder Stretch 2.

• Sit down at an area table and place your forearm on the table.

* Move the arm back and forward onto the table to allow the shoulder to open.

Repeat the motion at a 45-degree angle to the table.

* Next, slide in circles , if you feel comfortable.

* Repeat the process as many times as you like.

Shoulder Stretch 3.

Place your hands on the wall.

Then slide it back down when you are at a good height, Lean back against the wall.

* Put your hand back.

Repeat as many times as you like.

Rotator Cuff Stain

The rotator cuff is a part of the shoulders and it is comprised of tendons and muscles. If you've injured the rotator-cuff area, adhere to this procedure. You can also include the shoulder exercises mentioned in the above article and reverse the process.

Rotator Cuff Stretch 1:

Straighten up and place your arm a bit to your left and with your elbow facing at 45° to your left.

* With a straight-arm raise it about 90 degrees before bringing it back down.

* Make sure you are using controlled movements.

* Repeat the process as many times as you like.

Rotator Cuff Stretch 2:

* Sit on a chair , and carry either a stick or pipe at the palm of your hand.

The injured side will rest on the stick and the other side will take on most of the job.

• Place your hand on the side that is injured on the stick, then lift the stick using the other hand until it's just over your head.

* Slowly bring it back up.

* Repeat the process as many times as you like.

Rotator Cuff Stretch 3:

The exact concept as stretch 2. The hand that is injured is sitting down while the other hand does the work.

Then, place the injured arm's hand arm injured to the side of the pipe or stick and then use the second hand for pushing it toward the side.

* Repeat until you have completed the number of times you want to.

Rotator Cuff Stretch 4:

If you are still using the stick or pipe use your hand to hold the injured side at an angle of 90 degrees with your fingers in front.

Use the stick or pipe to pull the hand back. The motion is similar as the motion of the door closing and opening.

* Repeat until you have completed the number of times you want to.

It is also possible to use the term exercises for shoulder pain.

Knee and hip Strain

Hip and knee injuries can be caused by a variety of reasons, however they can be very difficult to treat if they're not addressed. Utilize the tips below to relieve any discomfort you may feel in these locations.

Knee and hip Stretch 1:

* Lay on the floor with your stomach facing down.

* Place your face on the ground , then wrap your arms around your back and grab your foot.

* Lift your leg off the ground. Your shoulder may be lifted off the ground too.

* Keep it for 30 seconds, and repeat 3 times.

Knee and hip Stretch 2.

• Lay down on the bed's edge. The injured side should hang off the edge of your bed. Make sure you don't fall off.

* Take the shin of your other leg and then pull it towards your body.

* This stretch lets the hip stretch with its natural weight.

* Stay for 30 seconds, then repeat three times.

Knee as well as Hip Stretch 3.

Sit in a chair while keeping your back straight. It is not recommended to lean towards your back during this stretch.

* Slowly lift your leg straight and slowly bring it towards the floor.

* If it's not too easy for you, consider adding the weight of your foot to increase your stability.

* Repeat 10 to 15 times, and increase the number as you gain strength.

Knee as well as Hip Stretch 4.

* While sitting in your chair, push your knee upwards.

* Slowly lower it. Be sure that your movements are in control.

* This is an exercise that strengthens hip flexion.

* Repeat this 10 to fifteen times. Increase as you become stronger.

Knee as well as Hip Stretch 5:

* Pick up an resistance band, then select the band with the one with the lowest resistance.

* Put the band across the middle of your foot.

* By using controlled moves, lift your knee and then press it down into the band of resistance.

* Repeat 10 to 15 times and increase your repetition as you gain strength.

Achilles Pain

It is the Achilles tendon comprises the muscle which connects the calf muscle with the heel bone. If we experience discomfort in this region particularly if it's persistent it's known as Achilles tendinitis. This routine will help heal this area and improve the condition of it.

Achilles Stretch 1:

* Begin by standing by the wall. You will have to lean against the wall.

* Stand up with one leg, and place another leg behind. The leg in front of you will be that is stretched out.

* Ensure that your feet are facing towards the wall and that they are level on the floor.

Bend your left front and lean forward into that leg, allowing it to move toward the wall. Keep your back leg straight.

* Stay for 30 seconds, and repeat three times.

Achilles Stretch 2:

* Sit close to the wall , and place your feet upon the walls.

* Place your feet as high as you are able against the wall, with your heel still in the ground.

* Lean against the wall using your body.

* Do this for 30 seconds, then repeat the process three times.

Achilles Stretch 3:

* You'll need an step ladder or step step to complete this stretch.

* Put the sole of your foot on the step, letting your heel hang over. Your other foot should hang off of the step.

* Lower on your heels as far as you are able to reach; you'll notice the tension in your Achilles tendon.

* Keep this in place for 30 seconds, then repeat it three times.

Back Strains

A variety of things can trigger back strains, from lifting heavy weights to having an improper posture or resting in a uncomfortable position. If you are suffering from a back strain, you should take this step to alleviate the discomfort.

Back Stretch 1:

* Lay on your stomach, then hold yourself up with your elbows.

Your hips should be at a level, but do not elevate your stomach.

* Keep the position in this way for 30 second, then repeat the position three times.

Back Stretch 2:

* This is merely one step up from the previous version.

* Lift yourself up onto your hands. Try to keep your hips on the floor.

* Keep this in place for 30 seconds, then repeat it three times.

Back Stretch 3:

* Transfer onto your back, with your knees facing the ceiling.

• Drop your knees down to one side and move your hips forward until your knees are touching the ground, begin rolling to the other side.

Repeat this 10 times, or hold it for 30 seconds, then repeat three times.

Back Stretch 4:

The following is the step starting Back Stretch 3.

* If you turn to the opposite side, drop your knee to the floor and then pull it up to 90 degrees and lower it down to the ground.

* If you'd like an even greater stretch in the lumbar area, hold your hands and place them on your upper leg.

* For 30 seconds, hold the position and repeat on the other side.

Back Stretch 5:

* Stand straight and put your hands on the hips.

Then, rotate your hips to look at the ceiling. Your hands placed on your hips should provide you some assistance. Don't bend your knees.

* Stay for 30 seconds, then repeat 3 times.

Chapter 5: Mobility Limiting Illnesses

Muscle and joint pains are usually caused by actions we take everyday However, in some instances the cause of pain can be ailments. These ailments usually manifest through no reason of our own, they're simply the result of due to genetics or age. Although there's not any way to prevent ourselves from developing the diseases however, there are things that we can do to lessen the discomfort to a great extent. These stretching exercises will reduce discomfort and help strengthen muscles and joints so that you can lead more at ease.

Arthritis

Arthritis is a common condition and is most often seen in older individuals however, it can be observed in teens or young adults too. It is the most frequent complaint on the hands and can result in stiffness and joint pain. Sometimes , it can cause swelling and redness in joint regions. It is possible that your mobility has decreased. If you suffer from arthritis, adhere to this plan to alleviate the stress on your joints and build your hands during the process.

Arthritis Stretch 1:

Place your hand on a counter or table. Allow your wrist to hang off the edge.

Warm your wrist by moving it upwards and downwards on your counter's edge. Repeat this approximately 10 to 15 times.

Change your wrist from side to side and repeat the motion ten to fifteen times.

Arthritis Stretch 2:

* Spread your hands as if you're showing the number 5.

* Make sure that your fingers remain as straight as you can and move your fingers one by one until they are in line with your thumb. This will allow the focus to be placed on the lowest joint of your fingers.

Repeat this at least three times over all your fingers.

Arthritis Stretch 3:

While keeping your hands open, put all of your fingers together, with your thumb facing upwards.

Keep your hands straight and straight. Bend the knuckle in order to create a 90-degree angle using your hands. Release the hand and return to straight hands.

* Then, focus on the joint above your Knuckle. Then, bend that joint inwards, nearly making

the appearance of a claw. Release it and return to the original position.

Then, shift to the top joint of your finger. It is also important to lower this joint it can be difficult, so keep your finger close to the joint, and then move it downwards. Make this motion by using both fingers.

Repeat each of these 10 to 15 times.

Arthritis Stretch 4:

* Begin with your hands open and your fingers are together.

Spread them large, and then bring them back to each other.

* Repeat this exercise for approximately 2 minutes several times throughout the every day.

* You can repeat the stretching exercises several times per day to alleviate any discomfort.

Tendonitis

The inflammation of the tendon can cause tendonitis. It is more frequent in some people more than other people. This is because of genetics or the pressure that is put upon the tendon. If you apply too much pressure or strain the tendon excessively it may cause tendonitis. If you are suffering from tendonitis on your heel, apply the stretching routine to stretch and stretching the Achilles tendon mentioned earlier. If you suffer from tendonitis on your wrist, you should follow the steps below.

Tendonitis Stretch 1.

* The first stretch of this routine is identical to the stretch for Arthritis Stretch 1.

Perform these movements, but make them slower and more controlled. You need to be able to feel stretch on your wrist.

* Repeat this 10 or fifteen times.

* As you gain strength and stronger, you can perform this using weight. You can try a soup container or something similar, and perform similar movements, however by holding the can.

Tendonitis Stretch 2.

* Spread your arm behind you, and then roll up your fist.

You can bend your wrist down and grab the opposite hand and pull it towards you.

* Keep it at least 30 secs.

* Spread your hands, then flip your wrists towards the upward direction.

* Use another hand and then pull your wrist towards you.

* Make sure to hold until you are able to hold for 30 seconds.

Three times in each way.

A different option is to place your fingers on the floor or a wall and lean against it all the way. You'll feel the stretch in your wrists, as well as the tendons that run up your forearms.

Tendonitis Stretch 3.

* Spread your hands until your fingers are spread.

Then, you can ball it into an fist. Repeat until you've done it as many times as you like.

* You don't have to hold it; the aim is to move your hand.

Tendonitis Stretch 4.

* Take an exercise ball or tennis ball.

* Press it with your hands for five to 10 seconds.

* Releasing and repeating five times.

* If you don't own an appropriate ball or need something that is softer, you can utilize a pool noodle, or a an up-rolled towel.

Tendonitis 5. Stretch

* Take an elastic band.

* Wrap it in your fingers and move your fingers to the side and close.

* Take it slow so that the band won't come off.

* You should repeat this three times.

Carpal Tunnel Syndrome

Carpal tunnel syndrome occurs in the wrist and arm and is caused by pinched nerves. The symptoms include sensations of tingling, sensitivity and the sensation of numbness. If you are suffering from carpal tunnel, adhere to this method of treatment to reduce pain and discomfort.

You will feel tension and stretching when you do these stretches, but without any extreme pain. It is possible to feel tingling on your fingers. When you release it you should feel it stop. If the tingling doesn't cease, it is an indication that you've overdone the stretch. The pressure is too high upon the nerve. It could also be a sign that something else is that is not right; this could be an ideal moment to consult your physician or your doctor to determine the cause precisely.

The Carpal Tunnel 1 Stretch.

* Put your hands to your face and close your fists.

* Lift your wrists upwards to make sure your knuckles are facing the ceiling. Then, bring them back to the floor.

* Repeat 10 times up and 10 times down.

* Move your hands towards the side to ensure that your thumb is facing upwards.

• Move the wrist upwards and down, using it is the same motion as previously.

* Repeat 10 times up and 10 times down.

* Make sure that you're making this an uninterrupted motion.

Carpal Tunnel Stretch 2:

* Spread your arms straight towards the front. Hands should remain wide.

• Turn your wrists up to point your fingers towards the sky.

* If you want to get less of a stretch put your fingers in a closed position. If you'd like to get more of a stretch put your hands on the wall.

* Keep it for 30 seconds, then repeat 3 times.

Carpal Tunnel Stretch 3:

* Keep your arms spread out before you. Turn your wrists to the side and then curl your fingers.

* If you'd like to have less stretch, then spread your fingers. If you'd like to have more stretch, place your hands against the wall.

* Stay for 30 seconds, then repeat three times.

Carpal Tunnel Stretch 4:

* Put your palms together in a prayerful arrangement.

Keep your wrists down while simultaneously your elbows must be extending toward the side.

* Pull as low as you are able to.

* Keep it for 30 seconds, and repeat three times.

The Carpal Tunnel 5 Stretch

* Hold your hands in front of you.

* Put your hands on the floor and then push your chest up.

* Stay for 30 seconds, then repeat three times.

The stretch is more of a peck stretch however, it's good for the whole region is connected, therefore it will still be useful for you.

6. Carpal Tunnel Stretch:

* Bring your hand to your chest at a 90 degree angle. Your hands should be the same height as your head.

* Maintain your chest in a relaxed position as you tilt your head to to the opposite way to your hand.

Repeat ten times. Repeat on the opposite side.

* This stretch is performed to ease the nerve out It isn't essential to perform it more than times per day, as it can cause irritation to the area.

4

Chapter 6: The Final Push Stretching Routines For Optimizing Your Training Routine

We have discussed the numerous benefits of stretching for your body and overall life. It can also increase the efficiency of your exercise routine as well. When you exercise your muscles are always moving and contracting. They are constantly in a state of motion. If you are not flexible enough and mobility, you'll experience a limitations in muscle movement. This could limit your training and speed.

It also boosts the speed of recovery following an exercise. When you stretch, you increase the flow of blood, which leads to more nutrients being available to the muscles as well as an easier removal of toxic waste. The end result is that you will feel healthier as a result of this. It also gives you a greater range of motion that means the actions that you perform are more fluid. Whatever stage you are on your fitness progress it is a great tool to keep in your arsenal to boost your athletic performance.

Utilizing stretching as a part of exercising is a great way to keep your body young and healthy. They can feed off each other. Stretching improves your exercise or workout and increases your overall well-being, and the cycle continues.

to get the most value out of Your Stretch

If you're an athlete or a fitness enthusiast, you'll want to be in a position to make the most benefit from everything you do. As with everything else, there's a right and wrong method to stretch. In order to reap the full benefits from stretching, it is important to be aware of a few aspects. The first is that stretching can cause tension, but not discomfort. The feeling of pain is normal. This indicates that you're utilizing those muscles. However, any discomfort or sharp discomfort is a sign that you need to end the stretch. It could indicate that you've done the stretching incorrectly or your muscles aren't prepared to perform the move yet. Flexibility develops with the course of time. Don't do it.

The other thing to keep in mind is that you need to take a deep breath. When we get concentrated on our exercise or stretching, we forget that we must breathe as we breathe in and out, muscles tighten up. Our muscles should be as relaxed as they can when stretching, so be sure to breathe in and out continuously.

The third point to be aware of when stretching is that it's not an exercise to warm up. Your muscles must be warmed up to make the most of your stretching. Muscles that aren't warm can limit movement and could cause injuries. The best method to get your muscles warmed up is to perform a five to 10 minutes of jogging, whether outdoors or on the treadmill. This will help activate your muscles and help them prepare to go on your daily routine.

The last thing to keep in mind when you stretch is to not be moving. It's about fluid movements that are not stop-start or pulsing movement. The amount of stretching is typically measured by the length of time you keep it for, not the number of times you stretch therefore if you're speeding up to reach the next stretch it will be difficult to achieve the maximum benefit from your stretch. Make sure to move as smooth as you can; also be sure to take a break and take in the moment.

Routines for Targeted areas

Each part of your body is unique, and when you're stretching, every part requires different needs and a different range of movements. I've broken down the stretching routines into segments and you'll be able to pair stretching exercises with the areas of your body exercising at the moment. In this way, you'll get the most benefit from your stretching exercise routine.

Following each exercise it is suggested that you spend a few minutes to be in touch to your body and participate in a state of mindfulness. This can be done by lying lying on the back, and breathing in deeply. Consider the way you feel and how the stretching affected the various parts that make up your body. It might be beneficial to rub the areas that you're considering physically. The aim is to strengthen the brain-body connection. If you are aware of your body, then you will be able to spot the details faster.

Upper Body Routine

Being a tight shoulders or chest that is tight will limit the range of motion you can perform, and you'll reduce the effectiveness of your exercise. Flexibility can help you

85

achieve greater results in every part that your body's upper. All of them are connected which is why it is important not to ignore stretching all over your upper part of the body. This routine will increase an increase in flexibility for your body.

1. Self-hug Stretch

* Relieve your shoulders. Hold each hand and place them on the shoulder of the opposite.

The arms of your body should sit above each other, creating the shape of a V around your chest. Your hands should be set further toward the side of the shoulder, not over the top.

Drop your shoulders as low as you are able to keep your eyes focused on you. Keep your chin in a downward position.

* Allow your chin to drop towards your chest until you're moving your eyes toward the ground. Your chin must remain in a tuck.

* The stretch should be felt in the middle and upper part of your lower back. Once it feels stretched, you should hold it for five minutes. Your shoulders shouldn't be moving as you breathe.

The stretch will lengthen the upper portion of the back. When your lower back appears straight, this can affect how your neck mechanics function This stretch can let this loosen up by introducing an arch that is slightly forward. A relaxed neck and back will lower the chance of injury when lifting weights.

2. Forearm Stretch

* Extend your arms straight towards the front.

• Flip your wrists up until your fingers point towards the ceiling.

* Grab one hand and pull them backwards. Repeat the same with the fingers of the other hand.

* It should be felt across your wrist, and the inside of your forearm.

* Keep it until you are able to hold for 30 seconds.

* Then, flip your wrist to the side and then bend your fingers.

* Using the other hand you can pull the hand curled toward you.

* You'll be able to feel the stretch running along the back of your forearm.

* Make sure to hold until you are able to hold for 30 seconds.

Repeat this three times for both ends.

The stretching of your forearms may be neglected, however this stretch is beneficial for both the forearms and fingers. Forearms need to raise and your fingers to flex to grasp. After a long time of not working the muscle of the forearm, it can get stretched and shrink. Many jobs do not require the use of the forearm muscles and it is our duty to ensure this muscle is in good shape, to ensure it is able to move.

3. Corner Pec Stretch

* Take a few feet from the corner of the wall. You'll need to alter the distance you stand according to your height as well as the arm length.

Place your palms each side of the wall at shoulder height.

* Breathe in and then , as you exhale, activate your core muscles and bring them back into your back Press your chest towards the wall, leaning against it using your entire body.

* Your body shouldn't be bent in order to perform this movement. Keep it for 30 seconds, then repeat the exercise three to five times.

* When you hold this position, it causes the chest muscles getting longer.

The stretching targets pectoralis major which is crucial to the way you position the upper part of your body. Instretched pecs can cause back pain because they aren't stretch enough they contract and pull your shoulders down. It is crucial to maintain good posture when exercising as well as in general. It is impossible to make the most of your workouts for the upper body in the event that you do not take care to take care of your posture. It is best to avoid this than to solve it once you are suffering from it.

4. Big Turn Back Stretch
* Look at a wall, and get as close to it as you can.
• Place your right hand in a straight line against the wall with your palm against the wall. The arm must be parallel to your body, and in line with the wall.
Begin slowly to rotate your torso left to right while your hand is still on the wall.
Stop whenever you notice a stretching in your shoulder and chest. Continue to build the stretch slowly, however, if you'd like to extend stretching, be sure to not push the stretch too far.

* Hold for 30 seconds, then repeat with the other side.

This stretch will open your chest, loosen your biceps and also loosen your shoulders. It will also have an impact in your posture. It will require the muscles in these exercises for lifting or pressing as well as any other upper-body exercises.

5. Wall Triceps Stretch

• Bend the left hand to the elbow. Then, place your elbow against the wall. Slide it upwards until it is higher than your head. Your hands should be in front of you, in the middle of your back.

* Grab your right hand, then grab your wrist to the left.

* Lean against your wall, and let it stretch.

* Keep it for 30 seconds, then repeat the exercise on the opposite side.

The triceps muscles are utilized to assist in extending and moving the elbow. It is also involved in keeping the shoulder steady. Your entire shoulder and arm will be able to relax and become more flexible if you perform this stretch.

We've all experienced an injury to the spine that causes it to click at some point. The popping or clicking is related to general joint and muscle function. There's nothing wrong with a back that is cracked however it could suggest that you haven't been stretching or working on your spine in a sufficient way. The spine is the anchor for the entire upper body, which is why we need it to be flexible and working properly. Stretching your muscles is an effective method to ensure that your spine stays supple and, if performed frequently, will relieve tension.

Thoracic Routine

The thoracic region comprises the region that extends from beneath your shoulders to your hips, which is your abdominal region. The thoracic region is home to twelve vertebrae , as well as your ribs. All your vital organs can be found in this region of your body.

When you workout muscles, they heal and then shrink, especially during are sleeping. The muscles that are shortening become stiff and can negatively affect your exercise. In order to ease this discomfort and allow you to be more comfortable to perform your next workout, you must stretch the thoracic area.

1. Cat-Cow

Follow the directions for the Cat-Cow Stretch in chapter 2. both the back routine and Torso routine in chapter 2.

This stretch has been proven to enhance balance and is a great stretch for all vertebrae. It also engages the tailbone to trigger the root motion of the spine. This lets the spine move more freely. If your spine is more flexible and has more mobility, it can reduce your chance of injury during various exercise routines.

2. The Cobra

Follow the steps on Cobra Stretch in chapter 2. Cobra Stretch under the Back and Torso routine in chapter 2.

Cobras are a spine stretch that can strengthen your spine. It's also great to stretch out your shoulders, chest and abdominal. Everyday activities can affect the health of your spine and spine working at your desk or carrying a child can cause our spine to curve to the side. This could affect us in many ways, including the fitness aspect, and this stretch can help counteract some of the negative effects that come from our daily life.

3. The Hip Hinge

Follow the steps for the hinge on the hip under Chapter 2. Back and Torso routine in chapter 2.

The act of bending is an integral part of our everyday life, which is why we have to build a strong core and lower back. It is essential for resistance training, deadlifts kettlebell swings and other activities which require an energised spine and lower back. This stretch will strengthen your spine and core , ensuring that you can move in these places.

4. Child's Pose

Follow the steps on the Child's Pose in the Shoulder, Neck, and Chest sequence in chapter 2.

Child's pose is extremely flexible in the sense of which body parts it can stretch out. It aids in stabilizing the spine as well as opening the hips and chest. There is a tendency to feel the backs of our lower backs compressed as we put extra weight into it instead of engaging the abdominal muscles. This posture can help us relieve the compression and make us aware of how important it is to engage our core muscles.

5. The Frog Stretch

* Get on your knees and hands.

• Turn your feet inwards to ensure that the inside of your foot is resting on the floor and move your knees out. They should be wider than your shoulders.

* Lower your hips to your feet.

* If you can slide to your forearms and lower them instead of resting on them, that will allow you more stretch.

* Keep it for 30 seconds up to 2 minutes.

This stretch targets the adductors and your groin and also concentrates on the core area, and that is the reason it's in this workout routine. If you've ever performed any form of exercise, or are an active person of some type you'll be aware of how crucial the core is to nearly everything you do. The muscles in your core are where the majority of your strength is derived, so having a flexible and strong core can help you perform better to perform any kind of exercise.

Low Back, Hips and Lower back

In gaining flexibility and mobility as well as strength in your hips and lower back is the best method to avoid injuries in these regions. Lower back and hip injuries are among the most prevalent in the world of fitness. In addition to preventing injuries, it is vital, but strengthening this region can help you achieve an improved lower-body workout and an overall body exercise. The area is located between your body and your torso and it is the one that carries loads of weight and stress due to daily activities and exercise. Do this exercise routine to strengthen your hips and lower back.

1. Supine Spinal Stretch

* Lay on your back, and then bring your right knee towards your chest.

* Grab your left arm and pull your right knee to cross the body . You will rest on your left side.

* Spread your right arm out to the side and then turn your head to gaze at it.

* Keep it for 30 seconds, then repeat on the other side.

This movement helps stretch your lower back, spine and also opens your chest by moving your lower part of your body in a way that isn't geared towards muscles and joints which are usually overlooked.

2. Seated Piriformis Stretch

* You should sit on the edge the chair, and keep your body straight.

* Grab one leg, then place your ankle over your right knee. Let the foot flex and then let it lie in line with the floor.

You can pin your leg by placing your hands on the ankle and your other on the thigh.

* Lean forward and pull your chest to your shin. Do as much as you can in order to increase the stretch.

Maintain your back straight throughout the day.

* Keep the hold for 30 seconds to two minutes, then repeat with the other side.

The stretch targets the glute, piriformis and hip joint and muscles. These joints and muscles are all essential to the movements in the lower area. You'll be using them when you perform exercises for strength or athletic training.

3. The Knight Stretch

Follow the directions on the Knight Stretch in chapter 2. Chapter 2. Knees and the Thighs found in chapter 2.

Knight stretch is a great way to open your hips, stretching the muscles in your legs. It also stretch your spine, and opens your chest. These types of exercises show how one movement can impact a variety of parts of your body. It also shows how interconnected your body is, and why balance between your mind and body is crucial.

4. Pigeon Pose

Follow the steps on how to perform the Pigeon Pose under the Hips and Glutes routine found in chapter 2.

If you are experiencing tight hip flexors that pull your pelvis backwards, and can cause negative impacts on the lower back. The lower back could be prone to an overly curved arch, and this means that in certain postures or movements, you'll experience discomfort. Flexing the hips by stretching them will assist in improving your back arch and allow you more flexibility while doing exercises.

5. The V-Sit

* Sit down on the ground with straight back. Keep your legs as wide as you can keep them.

* Lean forward using your entire body to reach for your foot. You might not be able to grasp your foot, then take your thigh or shin. Pull your leg downwards until you notice the stretching within your hamstring.

* For 30 seconds, hold the position and repeat the exercise on the opposite side.

This stretch will allow you gauge the flexibility in your hamstrings, as well as in that of your back. By stretching this way, it will enable you to enjoy more range of movement in your hips as well as an improved lower back.

Lower Body

1. Quad Stretch

Follow the directions for the Quad Stretch in Chapter 2. Knees and Thighs found in chapter 2.

The stretch is not just for just the quads, but the knee, hips, and the other muscles of the leg. It is particularly useful for stretching and strengthening your legs prior to vigorous lower-body exercises. Running, cyclists and even those who practice yoga often use this stretch to prepare for exercise and also help them cool down afterwards.

2. Hamstring Stretch

* Sit on the ground , with your legs straight towards the front and with your spine straight.

* Breathe in , and then place your body on your thighs. Then, reach to your feet. If you're unable to grasp your feet push as much as you can until you feel the stretching through your hamstrings.

* If you'd like more stretch then you can stretch your feet.

* Keep your hands on the floor at least 30 seconds. Then then come back and shake your legs. Repeat three times.

Hamstring stretching can help loosen the hamstring. As the result, it gives your body greater support. A hamstring with a string will provide your knees with more support while running or engaging in other activities.

3. Standing Forward Fold

* Stand up straight with your back straight and your feet separated.

* Bend your hips and move your body close to the thighs of your body as you are able. Make sure your knees remain straight as you reach out to the floor with your fingers. If that's not feasible then you should go for your ankles, or calves.

Try to move toward your legs every exhale.

* You must hold for 30 seconds until 1 minute.

This stretch helps to lengthen the hamstrings as well as strengthen your thighs and knees. There may be a feeling in your hips and calves and calves. This is a stretch that will work across your entire lower body.

4. Wall Calf Stretch

* Stand just a few feet from an unfinished wall.

* Move forward using one leg, leaving the other leg behind. Both feet must be facing towards the forward direction.

* Place your hands on the walls.

* Bend your knee the closest to the wall, and then keep the other leg straight.

* Lean against the wall using your body. Make sure your feet are to the earth. You will feel the stretch in your calf muscles of the lower leg.

* Keep the hold for 30 seconds to one minute, then repeat with the opposite side.

This stretch will not only work the calf and as well the Achilles tendon. This means there will be a more expansive range of motion as well as your leg as well as ankles will be stronger.

5. The Knight Stretch

* Follow the steps on the Knight Stretch in chapter 2. Chapter 2. Knees and the Thighs found in chapter 2.

Also, check out the notes below the hips and lower back exercise in this chapter.

5

Chapter 7: The Cool Down The Routine To Keep You Young And Healthy.

Stretching can have so many benefits and benefits, not just for your body, but for your mind and overall health. It's an excellent method to ease injuries and boost exercises, but it is important to not ignore the other benefits that go together. Overall, having good flexibility can improve your daily life. Being conscious of stretching can improve the quality of your living to a degree you'd never imagine.

The Routine

Before we begin our routines, we should concentrate on breathing and meditation as yoga practices however they go further than the basics. They are vital elements of stretching that can enhance your overall feeling after you're done with your routine, as well as throughout the rest of your day. They aid in connecting to our bodies and improve the amount of effective our stretching routines can be.

The significance in yoga lies in the fact that it doesn't concentrate solely on the body, but also on the mind well. The thoughts that go through our minds can influence the body, and that's why it's so crucial to be aware and capable of controlling our thoughts. This is where the practice of meditation is a key component; it can help us get our mind-body balance in the right direction. It assists us in focusing our attention on what's happening in our bodies and react to it effectively. The mind and the body are not two separate entities however, they function together. This is why they assist with daily movements and control of your mood that, believe it or not, do is not a major influence on the discomfort we feel in our bodies. The ability to stay aware of the state of your thoughts and body will bring you closer to your ideal life. It will also show in the responses of your body.

Breathing, we all know is essential in all aspects of life, but it's vital for stretching. If we are focused on breathing, our minds begin looking at our body; it can result in less chance of injuries. Breathing can increase oxygen intake. Our muscles require oxygen to perform at their maximum. Pay attention to the way you breathe in and out This can also be an effective tool to strengthen your stretches and decrease the stress that creates strain and knots.

Let's begin our stretching program. This exercise is great for strengthening your entire body. It was designed in the year 2000 by Winderl (2020). When combined with the meditation and breathing techniques we've talked about, it's an ideal combination for complete body and mind routine.

1. Standing Hamstring Stretch

Begin by standing straight and aligning your feet with your hips.

* Breathe deeply and bring your body to the hips. Then, grasp your legs' rear to the point where you can achieve it.

It is important to keep your upper back in a relaxed position.

* Pause for 45 seconds. 2 minutes.

2. Piriformis Stretch

* Follow the directions for the Piriformis stretch under both the back routine and Torso routine in chapter 2.

3. Lunge with Spinal Twist

Follow the steps to perform how to perform the Lunge With Spinal Twist stretch between the hips and Glutes sequence in chapter 2.

4. Triceps Stretch

* You can sit, kneel, or even sit down for this stretch.

Reach your arms out over you.

• Bend the arms to the elbow and reach the middle of your back by holding your hands.

* Using your opposite hand, you can reach out and grasp and pull gently on the elbow of bent arm.

* Keep it for 30 seconds, repeat on the other side.

5. Stretching and lying Figure 4

Follow the directions on following the Lying Figure 4 Stretching beneath the hips and Glutes routine found in chapter 2.

6. 90/90 Stretch

Follow the directions to perform the 90/90 stretch that are part of the hips as well as the Glutes exercise in chapter 2.

7. The Frog Stretch

Follow the directions on the Frog Stretch in chapter 4. the Thoracic routine described in chapter 4.

8. Butterfly Stretch

* Sit on the ground with your bottom feet in contact.

* Lean back and try to bring you head to as low as it is possible. Press your knees down by bending your elbows.

If your feet sit closer to your the more stretched will be.

* You must hold for 30 seconds until 2 minutes.

9. Seated Shoulder Squeeze

* Lie down on the ground Bend your knees, then keep your feet flat in the earth.

* Interlock your fingers behind you.

Straighten your arms. You will be able to feel your shoulder blades joining.

* Keep the exercise for 3 seconds and repeat between five and 10 times.

10. Side Bend Stretch

* Kneel down on the floor. Maintain your back straight.

Straighten your right leg and move it to the side.

* Put your right arm on the right leg of your body and raise your left arm into the air.

• Lean forward your body forward and turn your arms to the right.

Your hips must be straight ahead of you, with your right leg should be parallel to your body.

* Keep the timer between 30 seconds and 2 mins.

11. Lunging Hip Flexor Stretch

* Kneel on one knee.

* Lean in to the leg facing you, using your hips.

* If you press your butt and stretch it, it will give you a greater stretch.

* Hold for between 30 seconds to 2 minutes. Repeat with the opposite hand.

12. Seated Neck Release

* Sit or stand up with the back straight.

* Make sure your right ear is pointing towards the right side of your shoulder.

* Grab the right side of your hand, and gradually pull your head toward your shoulder.

* Keep the timer between 30 seconds and 2 mins.

13. Sphinx Pose

Follow the steps to perform the Sphinx Pose in back and Torso routine in chapter 2.

14. Child's Pose

Follow the steps on the child's pose in the Shoulder, Neck, and Chest sequence in chapter 2.

15. Pretzel Stretch

* Lay down lying flat on your right side. Place your head upon your elbow.

You can bend your leg on the left side, then move it towards your chest as is possible.

1. Bend your left leg inwards and then grab the leg with your free arm then pull it up so close to the butt of your body as you can.

* Slowly lower your left shoulder toward the ground, making sure your torso stays straight.

* Keep the position for 30 seconds and 2 mins. Repeat on the opposite side.

16. Standing Quad Stretch

* Stand up , keeping your back straight and your feet together.

* Bend your knees to the back, and then grab your foot using your hand. Bring your foot toward your butt.

* Make sure that you don't let your knees become separated.

* Press your butt to get greater stretch.

* Hold for between 30 seconds and 2 mins.

* Repeat on the opposite side.

17. Cat-Cow Stretch

Follow the steps for the Cat-Cow Stretch in chapter 2. both the back routine and Torso routine in chapter 2.

18. Knees to chest

* Lay on the floor with your back against the floor.

* Move your knees towards your chest.

* Grab your shins using your fingers and push them toward your.

Do not allow the lower part of your back slide off the floor.

* Keep the timer between 30 seconds and 2 mins.

Be a Healthier Person

Each part of your body functions independently. Everything is interconnected and works to benefit or harm of your brain and body. This is the reason why it is not appropriate to discuss stretching without mentioning certain other elements that are involved in conjunction with it to ensure you are healthy and content.

It is important to remember that regardless of the amount of stretching and exercises we perform, if we do not provide ourselves with proper nutrition, it could all be wasted. The foods you eat and the actions your body functions interact. This is the reason we have be aware of what we put into our bodies. It can be fueling us or drain our energy. Choose foods that are high in nutrients, select whole foods, and attempt to include fruits and vegetables into your diet whenever you are able to. You'll feel the changes in your body, your mind, as well as your energy levels. Vitamin B is crucial in your body's functions, such as the production of energy.

Sleep is an essential aspect of a healthy lifestyle. Many people do not think about sleeping, but it's the source of energy for the coming day. While we sleep the body heals itself and our mind adjusts itself in preparation for the coming day. If we don't get enough sleep or a poor quality of sleep, we deny your body of this ability to repair themselves and, before we have the chance to think about what our day is likely to be, we're already in a bind. If you get enough sleep your body will perform better. You will be more alert and take better decision-making throughout your day. Sleep is among my main concerns during training sessions with clients. And when you are working on your flexibility and fitness getting enough sleep is crucial.

Try biohacking and it will help you learn your own personal. What your body enjoys and dislikes, and the way it responds to different food and patterns. Biohacking is the process of making small adjustments to your lifestyle and daily routine in order to observe improvements in your overall health and well-being (Jewell 2019). The majority of biohacking involves trial and experimentation, and some call it split-testing, but it could help you understand the body you are in. Try an eating plan that removes something and slowly introduce it again and see what it does to your body or if you can add caffeine to your diet to boost increase in productivity and energy. Try sleeping at different times, or having an alternate bedtime routine, and note how this affects your sleep. The great thing about biohacking is that it could help you discover a way to live living a more fulfilling life that you did not know before.

When you are living an active lifestyle that is healthy creates an impact in your life that reaches numerous areas. Consider this: when you're well, you receive positive inputs and they will react positively with positive outputs and positive responses. Your body will be being grateful to you for less pain, and your mind is grateful for you with better control of emotions and fewer shifts. It will affect your thinking because you're more optimistic and positive, which creates more opportunities. You'll be more motivated to live a better life and contribute more. People like to surround themselves with happy people. This can greatly improve your relationships and enable you create new ones and stronger ones. It is important to remember that stretching can improve your mood too; when we stretch your body releases endorphins which can give us a buzz and improve our spirits. This feeling can last for hours after the end of stretching, and may affect the way you deal with things and the people who are around you.

The foundation of this healthy way of life is a balance between mind and body. This is vital because it's so crucial to be healthy in all aspects and not only in one area. If we concentrate too much on one area then we won't be stable and it will not be long before we collapse to the strain of whatever happens to us. Health is comprised of the pillars of body and mind and we must ensure both are healthy.

It's great to state that you require that balance. But the real problem is how to attain it. There are several actions you can take in your daily life to get you to an overall state of health. Move around and get up. Being seated for too long could have detrimental effects on your body and your mind. Make sure you do 15 minutes of heart-building activities every single day. Find something that feeds your soul. Consider asking yourself what is your greatest passion and then find an avenue to incorporate it into your daily routine. Give everyone a hug and give back. Also, make time to be present and an active participant in your surroundings. try to practice gratitude. The most crucial things is to be sure to laugh. The endorphins produced when you stretch will be released when smile. These are just one of the ways that you can get your body and mind in balance and any activity that brings happiness and peace could be added to the list.

There are many aspects to health, so make sure you investigate and pay attention to each one of them. Balance is possible by taking the right steps toward it. It's not a complicated or fantasy idea, but something that is accessible to all. It's your life that you live in, as is your body. you wish to live your life the best way you can. whatever you decide to do, make every decision now with the direction of the right direction.

Chapter 8: Warm And Cool

If you're planning to do exercises, it's a great suggestion to warm before and cool down once you've completed. If you do not practice this, you'll suffer injuries. The proper warm-up and cool-down include stretching, and in this chapter we're going to take a look at both of those aspects.

Start Off With Ease

When you make the effort to warm your body you'll experience greater blood circulation which makes it much easier for oxygen to flow into all of your tissues. The nerve impulses you receive are more rapid, which means that your muscles will be able to perform more efficiently. The process of warming up can also trigger an increase in your heart rate which means your cardiovascular system is capable of handling the stress that comes from your exercise. It's a great method to boost the temperatures in your tissue and the body in general so that you won't suffer injuries when you exercise.

If it weren't necessary to warm up before starting, today we wouldn't even be discussing it. The more comfortable you feel the more relaxed there will be in your connective tissues and muscles and the more easy it is for these tissues and muscles to grow more long, which means you'll be able to do the stretches with greater efficiency. You won't have to be concerned about causing injury to yourself. The disadvantage of doing your exercises or stretching routine not warming up is that you can easily get faint or dizzy because your heart rate is going up too quickly.

Three Stages

The warm-up routine you follow has three key phases. At the beginning, you'll start by doing the exercises you'll be doing later on, at a slower pace. In this way, you begin getting comfortable with the motion. For example, if you plan to cycle, it's a good idea to move your legs slowly, like you were biking. If you're planning to go for a run, begin with a quick walk first.

The next stage of warm-up is dynamic stretching. In this stage, you'll be doing complete body movements that don't need any connection to the training you're doing. The reason for these exercises is to allow you to extend your range of motion and allow you to traverse through the three of the three movements. They're fluid, rhythmic, and energetic.

After spending some time doing exercises like your workout, and performing dynamic stretching, you'll find that you're comfortable enough to add static stretching. This final stage of warming up can ensure that you're able to stretch your muscles, making it more comfortable for you to get your joints moving. The most ineffective method to start your warm-up is to do static stretches. Instead, start by practicing the moves you've been working on. then move on to dynamic stretching, and then end by doing static stretching.

When we speak of getting warm, we're not just about being more flexible. It's about trying to raise your body temperature at a temperature to move with greater ease of motion when you do your exercises. This means you shouldn't hang on to the stretch in the warm-up phase for longer than you would in cooling down. It is important to remain in your comfort zone so that you do not injure yourself.

Warm-Up Routine

If you're looking to get ready, you are able to choose the moves you'd like to do, so it is that they're like the exercise you're going to be doing. After you've finished this, you're ready to perform some dynamic stretches before you end with static stretches. Therefore, we'll review a few of these in a moment.

Dynamic Stretches

The Knee Lifts will allow you more flexibility within your lower back, back buttocks and hips.

1. Start by standing up with your feet in a row. Make sure your hands are to the sides.

2. Take a deep breath in. When you exhale then lift your right knee towards the chest.

3. Hold the knee in your hands and lift your leg up even more. The higher you are able to elevate your knees, the more you'll be able to stretch your hamstrings and buttocks.

4. Lower your leg back to its starting position, and perform the same exercise with the opposite side.

5. Repeat for 16 to 20 repetitions.

If you're feeling you urge to cheat and do something easier, simply bring your knees towards the sides instead of pushing them forward. If you're in the mood for a bit of test, you might want doing this exercise by putting your toes onto the ground. When you lift your body, you should raise your chest. must be able to exhale. Keep in mind that it's crucial to keep your shoulders down and your chest. Do not hold onto your kneecap as when you do, it puts stress on your knees and you might hurt yourself. Don't succumb to the temptation of bending your pelvis.

Core Twists exercise is great because your whole body will be able to feel it, particularly in your back, shoulders and abdominals.

1. Place your feet in a space that is distinct from the one. Lift your chest with your abdominals. Your shoulders should be lifted, then to your back, down and ensure that your hands are to your chest.

2. Breathe into your lungs. Let your knees bend slowly as you breathe out , and then pivot your right toe. While you are pivoting your shoulders, your hips should be turned toward the left. Make sure that your knees stay bent and your feet are spread. This is because you need your body's point of balance to be the lowest it can manage and

you'd like your upper body to feel comfortable.

3. The same procedure is done on the right side.

4. Repeat the stretch for about 60 to 20 repetitions. Be sure that your arms and shoulders remain in a relaxed position so that you can maintain the momentum of your hips as you move your elbows to the side.

The Chopper The Chopper: This is the exact move you'd perform when you chop the wood. It will feel throughout your abs, chest back, buttocks, and abdominals all at once. You should do this stretch if anticipate stretching, bending and twisting throughout your exercise.

1. Standing tall, keep your arms close to your sides, and your feet spaced hip-width apart.

2. Bend your knees at the knees. On the big toe of your left move your foot forward while lifting the heel of your left. You should have your left heel planted on the floor with your front facing forward.

3. Turn your hips to the left as you extend your arms forward and downwards.

4. Keep this posture for a long, deep breath.

5. Return yourself towards the center. Make use of the energy to push your hips towards the opposite side as you raise your arms above your head towards the right.

6. Maintain this posture while you take a long , deep breath. If you're doing it correctly the chest, obliques and the left hip flexor will feel it.

7. Perform six to eight additional repetitions of this stretch switching sides from one to the next. When you are stronger, you can do several sets of eight repetitions.

It is crucial to be mindful of your back spine when you perform this exercise Therefore, you should ensure that your hips move with you rather than looking forward throughout the movement. As you lift your arms upwards, take a breath in and exhale as you return your arms to the ground. Focus your attention on your spine while you do this stretch, and try the best you can to stretch it further. To ensure your back is safe it is important to keep your abdominal muscles in a tight position. Be sure that there's no Archer compressing your lower back. Also, ensure that your knees do not collapse to the side or bow. The idea behind this exercise isn't solely to depend on momentum, but to stay in control.

Static Stretches

We'll explore static stretches that will help increase your mobility as well as your muscles and joints. Remember, you're not looking to increase your flexibility right now, but you should ensure you're able to do the exercises. This means that you shouldn't do these postures for longer than you'd do when you're done your workout and then cool down.

Calf and hip Flexor Stretch The hip flexors as well as the your calf muscles are extremely linked to one another. If there's an issue in one, it could cause problems for the other. This is the reason you need to stretch both of them.

1. Keep your feet straight. Maintain your right foot as far as you are able to. Your heel must remain in contact with the floor.

2. The left knee should be bent while you lift the left arm up over your head, while pressing your hips upwards.

3. Clincher buttocks, so you can feel the stretching in your calf and hip flexor. When you push your hip forward and extending

your arm above your head, you'll be able feel as if your spine is lengthening but not compressing or getting shorter.

4. Keep the same position for 30 minutes, and repeat the exercise using the other leg.

Back and Hammies Stretch This stretch is designed to bring all the muscles in your back, from your lats all the way to the lower back hamstrings the heel, and calf. Make sure you don't hold an excessive tension on your shoulders, and make sure you aren't succumbing to the temptation of rounding your back when you do this stretch. This stretch is one of those situations where it's crucial to stay within your comfortable zone.

1. With a broad standing stance, keep your feet in a hip-width space.

2. Extend your right leg so that your left heel is on the ground and your right foot is pointed towards the sky.

3. Now , bend the left knee and tilt your hips slowly back.

4. Begin to reach your right foot by using the left side of your hand. If you'd like reaching for the side portion of your left leg.

5. Stay in the same position for 30 seconds, then repeat the exercise on the opposite side.

Make sure to maintain your back flat throughout this workout. It's beneficial to bring your hips forward.

The inner thigh and Groin Stretch This stretch can help your torso muscles. They will help you turn your spine and strengthen the muscles that make up the inner part of your thigh. Not only will they become stronger, but they'll additionally be more flexible. This means that you will be able to have an exercise that is free of injury and pain.

1. Start by taking a wide, stance standing up with all your feet pointed toward the outside.

2. Move your body forward slowly and extend your knees till your elbows just touching the inside of your knees.

3. As softly as you can manage, press your left elbow towards the inside of your knee. As you lower your left shoulder. Then, you rotate your spine to the right, while checking your right shoulder.

4. If you are tilting your pelvis, you should lower your hips by a further inch. If you're doing this correctly you'll be feeling it through your lower back. Imagine that your tailbone is begging to reach up for the sky.

5. In this position, you must remain for 30 seconds, then repeat the process on the opposite side.

Balance and Twist The stretch is an ideal one to try prior to starting your exercise.

1. With your arms to your sides with your heels together you can stand with good posture.

2. Change your weight to ensure that it is only resting on your left leg.

3. Lift your foot off the ground while making a an incline at your knee. Then moving all of your weight onto your left leg.

4. Turn your body to the right , and stay in this position for a couple of minutes. Reverse your body to the front. Make sure you are stable before getting to the twist. If you are struggling to stay balanced, you could utilize a barre or chair. Over time, you'll become more adept in this.

5. Stretch three times more.

6. Perform four repetitions on the opposite side.

Be aware that you don't need lift your foot far enough above the ground. There is only just a few inches between it and the ground. You must ensure that your hips are at an equal level. Should one of them be higher, it'll be difficult for you to remain balanced. Breathe in

Cooling Down

After exercising it is important for you to stretch out your muscles. This is known as the cooling down. It's an ideal opportunity to become more flexible since your body temperature is very high, which indicates that your muscles' structure are flexible. Since you'd like to improve your flexibility then you'll need to work on static stretches. These stretches will help you grow more supple within your muscle. In addition, they also lower the likelihood of feeling plenty of pain as you work out for hours.

We will walk you through an exercise routine that can aid in stretching your body from head to the toe. It can be done at home, or wherever you feel at ease. Remember that the majority of them will be done on the floor, which means you'll require a carpeted area or yoga mats. Take off your shoes prior to when you begin your stretches and remain hydrated. The more fluid you drink, the less sore you'll be.

Floor Side Extension The muscles that are going to target your obliques, and your waist.

1. You should sit on the floor and cross your legs the direction of your.

2. Reach your right arm over your head with your upper back muscles , so that your chest is elevated and your shoulder blade remains in place. There should be some space between your shoulder and your ear.

3. Breathe in and then as you exhale then bend your waist is moving towards the left, while your right arm is over the top. Make sure your hip is securely attached on the floor. If you require more assistance, you can place your left hand down on the ground. When you stretch your arms and turn your body you can imagine that your waist is getting longer.

4. Keep this posture in this position for 4 to 5 deeply and slow breaths, or for 30 minutes. After each exhale, you will go further to the point of stretch.

5. Repeat this stretch on the opposite side.

Back and Neck Extensions The feeling you get from this throughout your neck as well as your hips.

1. You should lie down on the ground. place your legs towards you, and then place your hands be on the floor. They should be on top and behind both of the legs. If you feel any discomfort or discomfort in your hips or knees while sitting on the ground, raise your hips off the floor with pillows, blankets bosu ball taking a step.

2. Breathe in, and as you breathe out, bend to the side at your hips. After each exhale, you will go farther into stretching by reaching to the front of your body with your arms.

3. Keep this posture for a while as you bring your chin on your chest.

4. Make sure there isn't any strain on your neck. You should shake your head like you're saying "no.

5. Turn your head to the left, and stay in the stretch and take several deep breaths.

6. Then, move your head to the left and stay in that position. Remain in the stretch and breathe deeply.

7. Get out of the stretch and stand up as slowly as you are able.

It's not necessary to have the same leg over the other. It's acceptable to swap the legs occasionally. So, you can ensure that your hips are in a good place. It is important to start the exercise by bending your hips, not from your back. Your chin should be down when you tilt your body towards the other side. Pay attention to your back and shoulders. It is not a good idea to put any tension or tension in them.

Butterfly Extension This stretch is designed to aid the muscles in your groin as well as your inner thigh.

1. Place your feet on the floor and maintain a an upright posture. Place your stomach in a tuck and ensure that your feet's soles meet. Your back should remain straight throughout this stretch since If you try to turn it around, it's going to create pressure on your spine as well as your lower back. You can feel your chest moving forward, and your pelvis pushing back.

2. Put your hands on the ankles while you pull your feet closer to your groin.

3. Take a deep breath in. While you breathe out and exhale, give the inner portion of your knees an easy push toward the floor by bending your elbows.

4. Keep this posture for 4 to 5 minutes of deep and slow breaths, or for 30 minutes. Try to keep them as far as possible.

Seated Hamstring Extension for most people, it's much easier to perform this stretch with the strap or towel.

1. Place your feet on the ground while extending your leg the direction of your body.

2. Bend the right leg to an angle that is comfortable.

3. When you breathe out then bend at the hips as you breathe out, and ensure your leg and foot remain in a relaxed position. Be aware of how your pelvis is moving. You should have the tailbone pushing forward when you move forward. If you're not able to connect your legs to your chest do not worry about it. It's all that matters is that you feel the stretching in your hamstrings.

4. Inhale deeply, taking deep breaths when you are there for 30 minutes. You can experience an even deeper stretch by lifting your chest while tilting back your pelvis, while making sure your foot is flexed to the side.

5. The same process can be done for the other leg.

Figure Four Twist, with leg extension: This exercise will strengthen your buttocks and core.

1. You should lie down on the ground. Your left leg should be extended to the side, then cross your right leg across you left leg. The hands should be in the air in front of you with your palms side down.

2. When the breath in comes, lift your left knee upwards and near your chest. Ensure the back of your body is straight to create an extended spine.

3. Move your spine to the side and gaze at your right shoulder, you tilt your pelvis back while you exhale. Pay attention to what's happening in your pelvis. If you're seeking a greater stretch in your buttocks or thighs, you should ensure you've got your abs and back stretched. Imagine that your tailbone is pulled towards the wall at your back.

4. Keep this posture for 30 seconds, then after each exhale, you will relax further to the stretching.

5. It's time to start working on the other leg.

This Straddle will strengthen your hamstrings back and inner thighs are going to be grateful to for this strap.

1. Put your feet on the floor and then extend your feet to ensure that they are straight and as far away from one another as you are able to get them. Your hands should lie behind your hips and you should ensure that you're sitting up at a height that is tall. Your hands are in the right place to maintain a an upright and straight spine and allow you to stretch without tightening your shoulders and upper back.

2. Your hips should be pushed forward not more than two inches or until you can feel the stretch in the thighs in your inner part.

3. Breathe in and, as you breathe out, tilt your head forward a little bit, with your pelvis in a downward tilt. Another variation of this exercise (if your muscles permit the) is to place your hands on the front while keeping your back straight. This will allow you to get deeper into the stretch.

4. Keep this posture for between four and five long and slow breaths or for 30 seconds, whichever occurs first for you.

Don't attempt to bring your chest on the floor if you aren't able to. This isn't the point here. What you're aiming for are your inner thighs.

You do not want a back that is round or your pelvis being tucked in.

Exercise your floor quads: Try this exercise for your neck, chest the obliques, back, and neck.

1. Place your feet on the floor to your left. Keep your knees near your chest. Then, place your head against your left arm. Check to see if there's no tension in your neck.

2. With your left hand, grasp the upper part the right side of your foot. Your ankle should be moved as softly as you can to close your buttocks. Do not force the motion to avoid damaging your knees.

3. Make sure you stretch your buttocks in a way that the stretch is more intensive. Pay attention to your hips. They'll be inclined to roll backwards, and you'll need to make sure they're on a level line when you move them.

4. Keep this posture until you've reached your 30 second limit. then turn to the right, repeat the exercise.

Your back as well as your Abs Stretch The more you work on these exercises, the more flexible your spine will be , and the less roundness in your back.

1. Lay on your stomach and ensure that your upper body is supported by your elbows. Your

elbows should be placed right underneath your shoulders.

2. Lift yourself up and outwards with your shoulders, so that you don't sink into your shoulder blades.

3. Inhale deeply and, as you exhale let your spine increase in length while raising your chest. You should feel as though your body is trying to move forward, however it's stuck on the floor between your elbows and hips. Your mind's eye can notice the space between each bone in your spine expanding and you'll feel it in your abs.

4. Keep this posture at least 30 seconds, or as long as it is necessary to breath deeply for four times.

The Wrist Extendment: This is a way of getting on four legs. If you suffer of carpal tunnel symptoms, don't try this.

1. Kneel down and hands. Your knees should be able to carry the majority of your weight.

2. Place the palm of your right hand down on the floor, keeping your fingers pointing backwards so that they face your knee.

3. Inhale deeply and, as you exhale gradually shift the weight of your body to your shoulders, away from your knees.

4. Maintain this position for 30 seconds, then be aware of the way your left forearm and hand feel.

5. Take a break from this position and place your hands back on the floor. Your fingers should point toward your knees.

6. Maintain this position for 30 seconds.

7. Try these stretches on another wrist.

Single-Knee Hip Flexor Extension If you are unable to do this on your knees use either a towel or cushion to ease your pain.

1. Take a knee and sit down.

2. Put the other foot down onto the flooring. The foot should be straight and straight ahead of you. The knee needs to be bent. Your upper body must remain straight. In the mirror, ensure that you're not having your back foot and leg bent in. If you're looking to feel this sensation in your hip flexor, make sure you place your hip ahead of your foot.

3. Take a deep breath in. While you breathe out then clench your buttocks, while bending your pelvis to the side. You'll notice that the sides of your hips begin to lengthen. If you aren't feeling this then try tucking your hips and tightening your butt a little more.

4. Maintain this position for 30 seconds.

5. The same procedure can be done on the opposite side.

Chapter 9: Full Body Stretch

Three essential things to be aware of while stretching your whole body. The first element that matters the most is your breathing. If you're planning to stretch breathing is essential as it's the way muscles become relaxed, which allows you to stretch further and make the most of the exercise. The best aspect of stretching your whole body is that you're able prevent yourself from becoming injured, and you'll learn good posture since the process of stretching involves maintaining your spine in a neutral position. That means you'll be able to keep your buttocks, hips and back over each other in straight lines.

We'll start this chapter with regular breathing. When you're breathing properly your stretch will be much more enjoyable and be more powerful in its influence on your health.

Breathing Right

The goal of this workout is to make you focus on your breathing. When you start your stretching, you'll be able to combine breathing with your movements so that there's no strain in your body. When you're doing it's recommended to keep your eyes closed all the duration. When you practice this, you're less likely to be distracted by your mind. This implies that it's much easier to be relaxed not only on your brain, but within your body too.

1. Lay on the floor, lying on your back, ensuring you bend your knees, and that your feet are down on the floor. Be aware of your body and ensure the spine remains in a neutral position to ensure that your natural curve to your rear is the way it's supposed be. Do not incline or pull your pelvis back.

2. Place your hands on the table and place your hands on the bottom portion of your stomach. then take an inhale by breathing through the nose. Let the air be absorbed into your lung. Take note of the way your ribs expand as you breathe.

3. When you breathe in and push the air out by your mouth. Or nose. Pay attention to how your ribs begin to shrink.

4. Repetition the procedure five times.

Floor Pelvic Tilt The more you perform this specific exercise and the more conscious you'll become of your pelvis and hip region. This area in your body will be the reason it is possible to climb stairs and maintain your balance when you move around. You'll feel it not only in your pelvic girdle, but also in your back.

1. Begin by lying on a floor that is carpeted or using a mat for yoga. Your back should be flat on the floor. Flex your knees and keep your feet on the floor.

2. Breathe into your lungs. While you breathe out then allow your pelvis to be angled towards the ceiling, to sense the feeling of your back pressing against the floor. There's nothing to worry about on your shoulders. The only body part that can be moving is your pelvis.

3. Return your spine to a neutral posture.

4. Do this stretching up to 10 or 8 times.

When you're doing this exercise, you must ensure there's no stress in the shoulders or your neck. Also, keep your upper back in the ground throughout the exercise. Additionally you're not working your glutes. So please not squeeze them as you raise your pelvis.

The Floor Arm Circulars When you do this exercise the shoulder girdle will appear more stable than normal. It will be easier to maintain your back in an upright posture whenever you move your arms around as well as an excellent stretch you can do prior to doing other upper-body stretches.

1. Begin by lying on the floor, with feet flat against the floor lying on your knees bent. Arms should remain at your side.

2. Inhale deeply, then lift your arms so that they're over your head, but they're still resting on the floor.

3. When you exhale then bring your arms back to your sides in the circular motion. Bring out your inner child and create a snowman.

4. Do this exercise between 8 and 10 times.

Bent Knee Spinal Twist: If your goal is to ensure you have an ample range of motion within your hips, buttocks and trunk, perform this stretch frequently. You must have flexibility in those areas since you will need these muscles for everyday activities.

1. Begin by lying down on your back, laying on the ground. Your knees should be dragged up towards the chest to ensure they are close. Your arms should be stretched out towards the sides.

2. Take a deep breath and, when you exhale then let your legs drop towards one end. As they approach the floor, ensure that your

arms are down on the floor. It's crucial to ensure that your head as well as your shoulder blade stay at the level of the flooring.

3. Keep this posture for 30 seconds and breathe in while you ease further into the pose.

4. Slowly and gently lift your knees back towards the middle, and repeat similar exercises on your opposite side.

A Floor Neck Stretch: If notice stress in the shoulders as well as your neck This is an excellent stretch to try. Take it slow when you do this stretch. It isn't a good idea to pull your neck muscles too much.

1. Place your feet on the floor and lie lying on the back. Keep your feet on the floor and keep the knees bent.

2. Lock your fingers together and put them on top of your head.

3. Breathe in deeply. While you breathe out gradually raise your head by using both hands. Bring your chin near your chest. Be sure to raise only your neck and your shoulders remain in the ground. If your shoulders drop out of the floor your exercise will not be as effective.

4. Keep this posture for 30 seconds and keep breathing deeply and ease further in the stretching.

5. Release the stretch gently and let your head rest on the floor.

6. Repeat this exercise three times.

While you're doing this stretch, be sure that you're not pressing too to hard on your head with your hands. Give the head a gentle push and that's all you need to do.

A straight hamstring stretch: It's require a chair for this stretch. This stretch can help to loosen your hamstrings which can be tight for the majority of people.

1. While your hands are resting on the seat in the seat, sit with your feet about hip-width apart. Your knees should be bent to the waist. Your knees must remain straight throughout this exercise.

2. Breathe in, before lowering your body to the chair.

3. Breathe in another deeply. While you breathe out and lower, you should do so by making your elbows bend while being supported by your chair.

4. Keep this posture for 30 minutes. If you ensure that your pelvis is pointed towards the

sky and your back is straight and straight, you'll see that there's an even greater stretch taking place at the back of your knees as well as your Hamstrings.

5. To rise from this position, ensure that you first bend your knees then slowly roll them up.

Intimate Thigh Stretch in Chair: If you're in search of an easy way to relax your back, shoulders, and neck this stretch is for you.

1. Take a seat and then stand on it.

2. The leg that you are able to towards the chair and place your foot on the seat. Make sure you are sitting with your hips and shoulders towards the front.

3. Take a few seconds to expel the air out of your lungs while you bend forward and let your hands fall towards the ground. Do not force the stretch. Instead, it's best to let gravity do the take over. If you're experiencing a lot of tension and strain then put your hand on the seat to gain more control while you move.

4. Every time you exhale gradually and slowly go further into your stretch. Keep this posture for 30 minutes. In order to ensure that you don't have any tension or tension in your

neck, move your head around as if you're saying"no. It should feel smooth and relaxed.

5. Relax and roll back up. Repeat your stretch again on the opposite side.

To make the stretch more effectively, it's a ideal idea to push your pelvis forward so that you feel the stretching in the groin. Additionally your arms and shoulders must be as relaxed as they can be. Don't attempt to stretch them to the floor with force. Let gravity do the work for you. If you're looking for challenging yourself, you could attempt this stretch with out the assistance of a chair or any other. In this is not only going to help you increase their flexibility in your quads you'll also gain stability. While you're performing this stretch, maintain the bend of your knee. While doing this ensure that you're standing in a good posture with your shoulders up and proud. It's not a good idea to bring your heel to the butt and it's wrong to pull your heel to the side of your hip.

Chest Extension Chest Extension: This is a simple stretch that can be done at any time. If you're someone who spends the majority of the day sittingdown, you should practice the stretch regularly. A few times per day isn't excessive.

1. Standing high and confident, and make sure your spine is in a neutral position.

2. Intertwine your fingers behind you. Your hands should rest near your butt. If it's really hard for you to keep your hands firmly tucked in to your back, use a small towel instead. You just need to grab each end of the towel with one hand.

3. Breathe deeply and, as you exhale then allow your arms to slowly straighten while you lift both hands toward upwards, off your back. Your hands should be lifted as high as you can while keeping your shoulders straight in your posture. If you're leaning over, then you've got an issue.

4. The position is for 30 seconds.

The Ground Hip and Butt Stretch The ground hip and butt stretch can be done this stretch from any location, it's better to perform it sitting especially if you're experiencing lots of tension in your muscles.

1. Sit in a chair. One leg over the other, and allow your ankle to rest on your thigh.

2. Breathe deeply as you place your elbow on knees within your part.

3. Breathe in as you lean forward and allow your spine to become wider while bending your pelvis.

4. Keep this posture in this position for 30 minutes, and then go further and deeper into the stretch as you breathe out.

5. Repeat this exercise on your opposite side.

Stretch, and ensure you keep your shoulders are at a lower level throughout. Lift your chest and allow yourself to breathe deeply in each exhale. Don't bounce or jerk and ensure you don't have your hip in a slant to the side.

Foot and Ankle Extensions If you can, do ankle circles throughout the day. This way, you'll be able to be sure you don't suffer an injury to your ankles since they're flexible and nice.

1. Place yourself in the chair. Check that your posture is correct and tall. Cross one leg over your left knee. Your ankle should rest on your thigh.

2. Hold onto the top of your foot using your left hand and hold your ankle with your right hand.

3. As softly as you are able you can, pull your foot back.

4. Stay in the same position for 30 minutes, and then release the position.

5. Then, grasp your toes using your right hand, and hold onto your heel using the left side of your hand. Slowly , begin pulling your toes back towards the shin.

6. Stay in this position for 30 seconds and then release it.

7. Then, grab your ankle with your right hand. Use your left hand to extend your hand beneath the foot and hold it towards the upper part of your foot.

8. Slowly and slowly, begin to move your foot toward the sky. Then, look around like you're looking for something under your feet.

9. Stay in the position for 30 second and then let it go.

10. Repeat these steps on the OTHER ANKLE and FOOT.

Tricep Extension and Side Reach The purpose of this stretch is to strengthen your back muscles in your upper arms.

1. Get tall, with a proper posture. Place your left arm above your head. Keep the elbow bent to your back, so that you can feel the tips of your fingers touching the shoulder's back.

2. Left elbow on left hand.

3. Breathe deeply. As you exhale take a moment to allow yourself to hold the left elbow slowly. Let it slide behind your head, allowing your fingers to move further back and reach your spine.

4. Breathe deeply and, as you breathe out, lean towards your right to the extent that you are comfortable. Don't twist.

5. Keep the same position for 30 minutes, and then return to the middle slowly until you release your arm.

6. You can shake your arms a slightly, then do the stretch on the opposite side.

Lateral Shoulder Extension will work on the deltoid's midsection.

1. Sit tall in a seat and raise your left hand. Your goal is for your elbow to be the same the height of your shoulder. Put your left hand on your right shoulder.

2. Your left hand rests placed on your right elbow breathe in as you pull gently towards your left shoulder.

3. Maintain the same position for 30 minutes, and repeat the process using the other arm.

If you'd want to, you can do this exercise while your arms are straight and not straight at your elbows. In this case all you need to do is extend your chest.

Chair Forward Bend This stretch is designed to stretch your back as well as the region that surrounds your spine. As you bend on your hips you'll begin be able to see that the tension within your muscles of the back can be easily released and the vertebrae may increase in length.

1. Place your feet on a sturdy chair. Get your abs in a tight position and make sure your feet are level on the floor.

2. Breathe in and , as you exhale let yourself stretch your hips forward. Stretch as far as you're able without feeling uncomfortable during the stretch, and allow your arms to hang toward the floor.

3. Keep this posture at least 30 seconds, or as long as you're able to take up to five deep and breathes.

4. You can roll back down and away from the position in a slow, steady manner and stack your vertebras into one another until you're standing high again.

When you do this exercise, you need be sure to start your exercise with your hips. Don't put your back into the exercise. You should also begin at your own comfort level and then gradually increase your effort to the next level, taking care to not injure yourself due to doing too much. Examine your shoulders and ensure that they're in a good position.

Wrist Flex (Standing) The stretch is standing. I've described how crucial it is to build the strength and flexibility of your wrists, forearms, and forearms. Here's the best way to do this stretch:

1. Keep your body straight and aligned, keeping your feet wide at the hips.

2. Straighten your arms and lift them until they're slightly out the front of you. Make sure you keep your hands on the hips and your palms facing each other.

3. Breathe in. Your thumbs should be rotated to the floor as if trying to move some knobs.

4. Continue to rotate until you have 30 seconds to go, but not more than you feel comfortable for you.

It is possible to find a more active version that is a more straightforward. Also instead of holding on to the position for 30 seconds it is possible to hold the position for several seconds, let go of your hands and repeat the exercise.

149

Forearm Extension Forearm Extension: This is a great option for those suffering from carpal tunnel syndrome. It will be felt throughout your wrists and forearms.

1. Get up straight. Place your left palm against your right fingers. Then, raise your elbows towards the sky.

2. Breathe into your lungs. When you exhale and out, gently press the fingers using the fingertips of your hand.

3. Keep this position for 30 seconds.

4. Do the exercise over again with your left hand.

Side Bends: When you practice this stretch, you'll begin notice it on your shoulders, back as well as your abs and the top of your hips.

1. Be tall, keep your toes facing forward and keep your feet separated from one another.

2. Lift your right arm over your head. Use the muscles of your upper back to ensure you can ensure that the blade of your shoulder is in the downward position.

3. Breathe deeply, and then as you exhale and bend your body toward the left. While doing this you can reach out and raise your body using your right arm to extend beyond your body. Place your legs into your hips until your

feet are level with the ground. Relax your left hand over the left thigh in case you need more support.

4. Stay in this pose during four or five minutes of deep breaths and slow breathing, or 30 seconds.

5. Relax gently and repeat your stretch again on the opposite side.

If you feel an increase in shoulder tightness Bend your elbow slightly instead of straightening your arm out.

Chapter 10: Strengthening Your Lower Body

Your lower body is deserving of just as much affection as your upper body does as well. If one area that is located in your lower back isn't functioning the way it should, the other parts of your body suffer just as badly. There are a myriad of issues result of tightness or tension in the lower part of your body, however it's easy to conclude they're the result of some other issue. From headaches to indigestion, the lordosis and scoliosis or even difficulties in breathing, lots of issues could be caused by an imbalance in your lower body muscle.

If you're a professional runner and you're not running with an extended stride It could be because you have tight hamstrings. It's inevitable that you'll need to take many more steps than someone who has loose hamstrings which means you'll have spend more time on the track, and you'll get exhausted faster as other runners. This also means you'll be taking on more force on your body that could result in devastating injuries. There's no better way to deal with this issue than stretching your lower body and also.

In this section, we'll review all the exercises you can do to your buttocks, thighs, and hips. You'll have an understanding of the pelvis's actions. The muscles that are involved in this exercise are linked to the pelvis and if your pelvis isn't placed in correctly it could be that your stretches aren't as efficient as they could be.

Buttocks and hips

If you're an active person, it's likely that you're experiencing an atrophic hipflexor that is tight. The hip flexors are known as the iliopsoas. They are composed of three muscles: the psoas majormuscle, the psoas minor along with the iliacus. These three muscles attach to the lower back region and run through your front pelvis and hips. Together, they enable for you to stretch your hips as well as move your lower back as well.

The more you exercise this muscle, the tense they become. Because of your hip flexors you are able to climb the steps and walk, run, or even move forward. They also assist you in being able to raise your knee whenever you need to. If you're spending the entire day sitting, you're bound be suffering from the hip flexors that are short and tight. Because they're linked to the lower part of your spine, it's natural to experience some pain in the region.

Let's discuss your glutes. They're one of the most important muscles in your butt. It's comprised of three muscles that include the gluteus maximus, the gluteus medius, as well as the gluteus minimus. The gluteus minimus acts as the hip abductor. It makes it possible to rotate your thighs inward and backwards. The gluteus medius is a middle-sized glute that aids you in shift your leg towards the side. It is a part of your gluteus minimus muscles to help you move your thighs forward and backwards. The gluteus maximus muscle is the largest and most powerful muscle in the butt. They aid in the extension of your hip and also rotate it.

Your piriformis is an important muscle that keeps your spine level. It is working, along with the muscles of the iliopsoas to provide equilibrium in your pelvis. When one of these muscles is fragile or tight, you may have issues with your posture and you feel lots and pain throughout your low back. This is why you must keep the range of motion and the strength in these muscles. You should aim for the right balance between flexibility and strength between your piriformis, your glutes, buttocks and the iliopsoas muscular. Therefore, we'll review some stretching exercises that will assist you to achieve this.

The Runner's Lunge stretch is a must for anyone, not just for runners. You'll be feeling this stretch in your iliopsoas as these muscles are vital for back health and the health of your legs as well. The stretching of this muscle shouldn't be an option , but rather it should be a requirement. If you are trying to perform this stretch and experience an uncomfortable sensation, it's an excellent suggestion that you keep the front of your foot on the floor and to keep the back of your leg extended. You can rest your back on a bench to support it.

1. Begin by standing. Maintain your legs at least two feet from each the other. Place your left foot forward and your right one behind.

2. Inhale deeply and then as you breathe out then flex your knees until they are bent to the side, then you can place both your hands on the ground directly in front of your left heel.

3. Now, you'll want to move your right leg as far as you can in order that you are able to drop down to your knees on the floor without feeling as though your kneecap has been bearing too many pounds.

4. Maintain this posture until you can take four or five minutes and slow breaths, or 30 seconds.

5. Do this stretch to the left.

Be sure to are kneeling at 90 degrees as you do this stretch. Also the knee must be directly aligned with your toes. If your knees stick over your toes then you're in trouble. Be cautious since if you don't you'll hurt yourself. Ideally you'll want to do this stretch and the other ones in this book the mirror, to ensure that you are aware of whether you're doing it correctly or incorrectly. Whatever you choose to do, you shouldn't let your kneecap to take on all of the burden. Move the weight towards the part of your leg right above your knees.

Floor Glute Stretch using the foot to shoulder: This is the ideal stretch for you to focus on the gluteus maximum.

1. Lay on the floor lying on the back. Make sure your legs are fully extended the front of you.

2. Make sure that your right knee is to your chest and ensure that your left foot remains straight.

3. Place the top of your knee with your right hand, and then your right ankle is on the left.

4. Breathe into your lungs. While you breathe out, bring your foot closer to your

opposite shoulder. Keep your knee in mid-section of the body. Be sure your shoulders and head are at the same level.

5. Maintain this posture for four to five minutes and deep breaths, or 30 seconds.

6. Now, you can stretch the opposite part of the body.

If you'd like to do this, you can do it in a sitting position with your back to the wall. Be aware, however that you should ensure that your back is straight and your opposing leg stays straight. While you're stretching ensure that you're not pulling just your foot. If you do you'll put a plenty of stress over your knee. Make sure that your pelvis doesn't get being pulled down. Instead, imagine moving your tailbone toward the floor.

Glutes Stretch: This specific stretch will hit the nine muscles in your glutes with ease. If you have an achy buttock and piriformis, this could cause the sciatic nerve to become squeezed, and you'll experience discomfort similar to sciatica.

1. Start lying on your back with your feet set flat on the ground with bend your knees.

2. Then, lift your left leg and place it to the left ankle , above the top of your right leg. The best position is above the knee.

3. Lift the right foot off the floor and inhale as you exhale. Let your knee pull towards the chest with both hands. Make sure you keep your fingers locked behind your right knee, so you are able to provide assistance. If you don't feel at ease to lock your hands, simply use a towel, wrap it around the rear of your thigh, and gently push toward your chest.

4. Utilizing the elbow of your left, provide the left leg a soft push away from your.

5. Keep this posture for 30 seconds and then continue to increase the intensity of your stretch each time you exhale.

6. Switch legs, and repeat the stretch over and over.

The Rotator Cuff Flex (Sitting) If you perform a lot of dancing and dancing, this is a beneficial stretch that will give you more motion within your hips and thighs.

1. Place your feet on the floor and stretch your left leg to the side. Place your right foot on you left leg.

2. When your breath comes in, extend the right leg a soft pull to your chest using the left side of your hand. Make sure you're sitting in a straight position. If you find it helpful, imagine that it's like you have a string attached at the crown of your head, and it pulls you up and causes your spine to lengthen.

3. Keep this posture for 30 seconds before continuing to deepen the stretch with each breath and exhale that you take. If you're doing it right you'll be able to feel the stretch in your back, which is why you must pay close focus on how you place your pelvis. Assume that another string is attached to your tailbone. Then it draws your tailbone close to the wall that is behind you.

4. Change sides and repeat the stretch.

It's also important to avoid putting your pelvis beneath you and also ensure there's no rotation happening with the back muscles. Maintain your back straight as much as you can and ensure that your spine is straight and straight prior to doing the rotation. If you're trying to show love for your neck muscle it's recommended to check your shoulder. Be sure you've placed your knee in close proximity to your chest prior to getting to the dormancy.

Focusing on the Back of Your Thighs

When you must stretch your hips or bend knees there are three muscles that aid you accomplish this task:

* The biceps femoris biceps.

*The Semitendinosus.

Semimembranosus.

They are commonly called the hamstrings or "the Hammies." They're located at the rear of your thigh in close proximity to each other. When you walk you must use your muscles called hamstrings. If you've suffered any injury to them it's extremely difficult and will take a long time them to recover. Additionally, it's frequent to see old injuries occur and cause additional problems later. Instead of and waiting around for your injury to occur prior to taking care of the muscles, it is best to be vigilant about protecting them.

Hamstring pulls aren't jokes. These serious injuries can be result of tension. When you stretch your muscles to the limit or contract them too quickly, it could be due to an imbalance in power between the quadriceps as well as your muscles in your hamstrings. There could be a difference in imbalance in strength and balance between your right and left legs. The majority of the time injuries are the result of an inflexibility within your legs. If you ensure that you have hamstrings that are flexible, you won't need to be concerned about the possibility of this injury occurring to you.

Floor Leg Extensions The floor leg extension is the most simple position to perform that can help your hamstrings remain isolated, without affecting other muscles. If you're confident that your hamstrings are tight it is possible to utilize a strap for stretching or towel to help you do this stretch. Your upper body needs to be as comfortable as it can. If you're feeling muscles that are tight in the upper part of your body you're doing something incorrectly.

For hamstrings that are extremely tight it's best to do this stretch while in a hallway with one foot on the floor, and the other positioned against the jam of the door. As more flexible and flexible become in your hamstrings, the more easily you'll be able to lower your hips towards the wall.

1. Begin by lying down on your back with your feet straight to the ground. Keep them closer in your buttocks to where they can do.

2. Lift your left leg and extend it to the sky.

3. Place your hands behind your thigh, and the hand behind your knee or behind your calf.

4. Breathe in, and when you breathe out then let your legs push towards the shoulders. Be sure to ensure that your shoulders are in the same position on the ground. As you exhale, each time you will notice the stretch getting more and deeper until you reach the point at which

it would be uncomfortable to move any more.

5. Stay in this pose for between four and five minutes and long breaths.

6. Repeat this stretch on another leg.

When you stretch be sure to feel it on the rear side of your leg. Don't try to meet your requirements, or even your nose, since this isn't the goal in this exercise. That being said, ensure your hips are firmly connected in the direction of the earth. Do not tuck your pelvis below and ensure that you don't have any the back of your head is rounded. The main thing you should be concerned about right now shouldn't be how low you're able to get your leg. You should feel your hamstrings stretching.

Standing Chair Stretch If it's not practical or comfortable to stand on the ground it's a great stretch you can do. You'll need an armchair or bench or perhaps an interior wall. Make sure that no matter what surface you choose that your foot isn't coming upwards higher than your hips.

1. Make sure you stand straight and with a good posture, and keep your feet down on the floor while your abdominals are lifted.

2. The left leg should be raised and place your chair on bench right in the front of you. Be aware of your hips, and ensure that they're straight. They should be facing forward and your legs should be straight.

3. As you press in, and breath out, bend your hips until you can feel the stretch coming from the rear part of the thigh. Take note of your back, and ensure that you're not overextending it.

4. Maintain this position for 30 seconds.

5. Do the same with the other leg.

If you're trying help an area of muscles to relax, it's a great option to engage the opposite muscle group. The quadriceps are the muscles that you contract, and they are the muscles that are located in on the sides of your thighs. Also you stretch your hamstrings to the rear on your lower thighs. This way, you'll be able to feel your hamstrings relax more as you stretch them, and you will be able to go further into the stretch to get maximum outcomes.

Hurdler Stretch (Modified) Hurdler Stretch (Modified) main issue with the original stretch is that it is painful for knees, therefore this is an improved version that will keep you safe. Another advantage of the stretch is it will be exercising your back and calf muscles too. If it's helpful with your stretch, try using an elastic strap or towel.

1. Place your feet on the ground and keep one leg stretched towards the front. Turn your right leg towards an inside angle, making certain that it's at a good angle. Your arms should be in your thighs.

2. When you exhale and breathe in, bend your hip, making sure your left leg stays as straight as you are able to keep it and that your foot isn't in any tension it. If you notice that the left leg is leaning slightly or your back is getting more tight and tense, it is a sign that you've gone too far. Try dialing back. If it does help then you can imagine that there's a string on your tailbone that pulls you toward to the wall

behind, and another one that's connected to your heel which is pulling it towards your front wall. In this way, you'll notice the back of your legs expanding across both sides. It is helpful to also have your tailbone all the way back it is possible to reach when you bend your hips.

3. Maintain this position throughout 30 minutes, making sure to breathe deeply both in and out. If you'd like to get further into the stretch each time you exhale, you could lower your pelvis even further then raise your chest and then flex your foot until you keep your feet moving towards your shoulders.

4. Perform the stretch again and repeat on the second leg.

In some instances you'll notice it's difficult for you to maintain your neck or shoulders in a relaxed position. If this is the case, you can use a stretching strap or towel to secure it to the foot's ball. Once you've got it secured and comfortable, gently pull the two ends of the rope or towel.If you feel that your chest doesn't seem to get near towards your leg it's crucial that you feel the stretch on the back of your thighs that means you're performing a great job. When you stretch ensure that your eyes are directed towards the floor, right behind your toes.

The Quads

The quadriceps, also known as quadriceps, and all muscles located in front on your thigh. They all work together to allow to walk. The muscles involved are:

* The rectus femoris.
* The greatus lateralis
* The medial vastus
* The greatus intermedius

Their primary function is to aid in the extension of your knee. That means that you work the muscles frequently when there's a lot of tension and tension in them. It creates an uneven tension on your muscles and can cause excruciating knee discomfort. We'll stretch to ensure you achieve flexibility in your quads.

Lateral Quad Stretch To do this stretch, you'll need to lie on your back. The benefit of this exercise is the fact that it's extremely simple to keep in the correct posture when you're used to it. Also, this stretch is great for those who are new to the sport.

1. Start by lying down on the left, with your knees bent and your legs close to your chest.

2. Keep your right arm in the bent position as comfortable as you can under your head. It is important to keep the arm resting on your head.

3. Stay on upper part on your left foot and then let your ankle gently pull toward your butt. Your quads will begin to stretch. The stretch will get even more intense when you tighten your buttocks. However, be careful, making sure your hips don't slide back. It's a good habit to ensure that your hips are in alignment with each other as you direct all your energy toward pulling your knee back. Don't make your heel touch your butt. If you do you'll put lots of stress on your knee.

4. Keep this position for 30 seconds.

5. Do this stretch using your left leg, lying onto your back.

It's common to elevate your knee when you do this stretch however this isn't a the best way to perform it. Make sure to keep your knees in contact with one with each. Keep breathing. Don't try to force your foot toward your butt. Also, keep your lower knee bent to ensure you stay in a good posture. If you're looking to get more value for your money place your pelvis on the floor.

The heel to the glutes (Face down) Face Down: If you've done a vigorous exercise and are feeling a bit sore in your quads This is a great stretch that can be added to your cooling-down routine.

1. Begin by lying down on your back. Maintain your face lowered and your legs spread towards the back. Make sure that your right hand is on your side.

* Make a fist using your left hand and then lift your head. Utilize your fist to help keep your forehead in place.

* Using your right hand, reach backwards and secure the upper part of your left foot. Make sure that your foot is in the right the position you want it to be. If you

are finding it difficult to hold your foot, simply hold onto your ankle at the side the heel. It is also possible to grasp the bottom of your trousers. The last thing you want to do is to forcefully push downwards on your foot. Instead, allow your foot to relax into your hands and focus on pressing your hips closer to the ground. So the stretch will focus on your quads, and will not put stress on your knees.

* Take a long, deep breath and then while you breathe out then give your buttocks and thighs an easy squeeze as you gently press the hips into the floor. Be sure to not let your right knee be pushed to one side as you reach to it with your left hand. It may be difficult, but you must keep your knees near each otherso that you don't have any misalignment and consequently, there's no chance of straining your knees.
* Hold this position for 4 to five slow and deep breaths, or for about 30 seconds.
* Repeat this stretch on the opposite leg.
The knee to Glutes Stretch This stretch is great for strengthening your quads.

Because you'll have to perform the stretch on feet, it's practical and simple to stretch after exercising outdoors since it doesn't require lying on the ground.

2. Make sure you stand up in a good position and place one hand down on a smooth solid surface. You could make use of a fence, a entranceway, a wall an armchair, or whatever to keep your balance.

3. Breathe deeply and elevate your right knee toward the sky. Secure your right ankle or the upper part of your foot with your left hand.

4. While you breathe in and breathe in, slowly lower your right knee and then gently move your right foot closer to your buttocks on the right side. It is important to ensure that the insides of your thighs meet each other , and that your focus is to move your knee backwards. If you're looking to do this stretch it's best to put your pelvis underneath and envision that you're tailbone advancing towards the floor.

5. Do this for at least 30 seconds , or between four and five deep, long breaths.

6. Perform the stretch on your other leg.

If you're hoping to let this exercise work for your balance, it's a great idea to avoid holding your feet to the flooring and see whether you are able to maintain your balance when exercising your quads. Make sure that as you do this exercise, you put your app into. Then, lift your chest and make sure your shoulders are in the right direction, and you'll be able to feel the stretch well. Don't try to make your foot touch your butt. You'll also observe that your knees are likely to want to shift towards the side. Avoid this by making sure that the inner portions of your legs are connected to one another.

Stretching Your Thighs In The Inner Parts of Your Body

Your groin contains five muscle groups: pectineus griscilis and adductor magnus. They also have the adductor brevis and adductor longus. I'm not sure that it's going to be simple to remember these terms even if you're not a physiotherapist , doctor, but we'll just refer to them as your inner thigh muscles, or your adductors.

These muscles are required whenever the legs move. They're as important as the muscles in your hamstrings. If you've got tight adductors, it's likely that you'll suffer from injuries. The worst thing you could happen is to be forced to treat injuries to the thighs in your inner thighs as it's a very awkward region regardless of whether your doctor is an expert and does this for an income. The best method to avoid worry about injury is to ensure the muscles are as strong as they can be and to stretch them frequently to keep them flexible.

Groin Stretch Groin Stretch: There are a myriad of stretch exercises that you can perform to help make your adductors more flexible. But, this is likely to be among the most effective ways to stretch your entire groin region without causing the tension on your neck, shoulders or back. A tip to follow is to work in an exercise chair to do this stretch.

Additionally, the chair needs to be strong, so that you don't get smashed.

1. Sit on the chair, and raise the nearest leg to allow you to set your foot on the chair. Your hips and shoulders should look forward.

2. Slowly, lean to the side while you exhale and then lower your hands down to the floor. Do not try to force the stretch, let gravity to play your part. If you notice excessive tension or strain being created, it may be beneficial to put one hands on the chair so that you have more control over how much you extend.

3. Gradually, and gradually go further into your stretch, exhaling each time you breathe while remaining in the position for 30 minutes. To ensure there's no strain in the neck area, you can try moving your head in a circular motion like you're saying no.

4. Slowly rise from the posture and return to upright. Then repeat the stretch on the opposite side.

If you're looking to feel this sensation in your groin area, it's best to pull your pelvis back.

The Floor Straddle Stretch In light of the amount of time spent on this stretch and how difficult it is to perform in a proper manner. It is important to ensure that your back and your inner thighs and your hamstrings are functioning as one, to ensure that you are able to perform this stretch correctly. If you experience tightness in any of these areas that you are in, the odds of a stretch working for you is slim to none.

1. Place your feet down on the ground. Make sure your legs are to the front of you. ensure you're feet as separate from one another as they can be.

2. Set both hands behind your hips. Sit up to the highest height you are able to. When you set your hands in this manner your spine is left with no other choice than to stay straight and straight, and then lift it. By keeping the hands in that posture will allow you to stretch your thighs back, hamstrings, and back without creating

tension that isn't needed in your back or shoulders.

3. Now is the time to change your hips. Move them forward several inches until you begin to feel the stretch on the inner thighs of both.

4. Inhale deeply and out. As you exhale move your pelvis forward slightly, tilting your pelvis back.

5. Maintain this posture during four to five long breaths and slow breathing, or for 30 minutes.

If you're having trouble finding it difficult to keep your back straight and also to move your hips forward, it's best to do it while sitting lying on a cushion or on the floor on a towel or blanket. When your hips are lifted off the floor the strain that you experience in the hamstrings be reduced significantly, meaning you'll be able to focus on your thighs' inner thighs more attentively.

As you perform this stretch, be sure you keep your knees with your toes with your back to towards the ceiling. It is important to ensure that your chest is elevated. Your pelvis is tipped towards the back. Breathe as deep as you can throughout this stretch to ensure that you can ease further into it, preventing tension from forming in your muscles. There is no reason to place your hands on the floor on your hips unless you plan to keep them there, while avoiding letting your back sway out or your pelvis pulled into.

Stretching the lower legs and feet

Your calf and shin form the lower leg. The calf is home to a lot of muscles, however there are two muscles which you should be aware of. The muscles that are concerned include the gastrocnemius as well as the soleus. The gastrocnemius provides the calf definition while the soleus sits under the gastrocnemius. They are muscles that you utilize when you push your feet towards the ground or push it off as you jump, walk, or run. An Achilles tendon connects the muscles and your heel. If you find that your Achilles tendon is a bit tight, it could cause strain on your Achilles tendon which isn't a great thing.

Calf Stretches: When you are constantly standing or wear high-heeled shoes every day You'll notice that your calf muscles shrink and become tighter which can cause lower back discomfort. This stretch is perfect for you. It's best to identify times during the day that you can do a few repetitions.

1. Place your feet one foot from a solid wall or surface. Be sure to face the wall, and ensure that your feet are together.

2. When your body leans forward make sure you place your hands directly against the wall.

3. Retract your right foot as far as you feel comfortable for you and leave your foot on the floor.

4. While keeping your left knee straight, you should have some slight bending towards your left knee. It might feel odd, but try the best you can to ensure that your feet are to align to your heels. If your toes are allowed towards the outside, you'll not benefit from this exercise.

5. As you exhale, when you exhale then gently pull your hips up. Be sure to ensure that your right heel is in the ground.

6. Keep this posture for a few minutes and then bend the right knee a bit, without lifting the heel off of the ground. The knee bend is vital since you're working muscles that help by flexing your ankle.

7. Do the same stretch on the opposite leg.

One-Knee Achilles Stretch: If your never had an injury or rupture to your Achilles tendon in the past then, make sure you don't ever. This is a terrible injury and is best treated by surgery or complete immobilization with a cast for a prolonged time. It's much more comfortable for you and your financial account to ensure that the area of your body is healthy and flexible throughout the day and a great method of doing that is to stretch frequently.

1. Kneel down by pushing your hips forward onto your heel, while the other foot is in a flat position near the knee.

2. Place your hands forward on the ground , and breathe into your lungs. When you exhale then allow your weight shift upwards. Make sure you are able to keep your heel on the floor and leaning towards the front. When you reach this point you'll notice a stretch in the Achilles tendon that runs along the front of your leg.

3. Maintain this posture for four to five minutes and slow breaths , or 30 seconds.

4. Repeat this stretch for the second leg.

Shin Stretch Shin Splints, or another horrendous injury to sustain. They result from exercising on the hard surface, overusing your muscles and not being flexible enough and having fallen arches within both of your feet. This stretch can help to ensure that you do not to suffer from that injury.

1. Kneel down on a mat or carpeted floor. Make sure that your feet are pointing backwards.

2. Begin by gently lowering your hips until they are on the floor, and then sit upon your feet.

3. Breathe deeply, and then as you exhale then grab the top of your left foot and gently pull it towards your butt. There will be a stretch in the left shin.

4. Keep this posture for a short time and then let your muscles.

5. Perform a few repetitions more on the right. move to the opposite one, taking care that that you perform the same amount of reps on your left side.

If this isn't a good posture your body, or if you have an excessive amount of knee pain due to the fact that you don't have the same flexibility, you can roll a towel , and put it behind your knees, under your buttocks. A second thing to consider is that you'll require a rug or mat that is comfortable as you do this stretch. Although it may feel slightly tight at the beginning, keep in mind that it's fine to sit in your heels. To maximize your performance, you must elevate your abs while you lift your foot, and maintain your spine in a neutral position. If you're sitting on the ground instead of sitting on your heels it's not going correctly. If you're sitting in between the heels of your feet, you'll place strain on your knees.

Heel Stretch The feet perform lots of work when you walk, run and leap. If you're looking to improve your performance and improve your performance, you need to make sure your feet and ankles aren't tight and rigid. This stretch is designed to strengthen those muscles in the foot's bottom.

1. Begin on all fours using your knees and hands on the ground.

2. Move your feet to the point that your feet are in the direction of your knees.

3. Breathe inand let your hips return and lower to the heels while you push your heels closer to the hips. You'll be able to see this stretch frequently in the lower part of your feet.

4. Continue for 30 seconds as you breathe deeply. Each time you exhale, you should continue to stretch deeper in the stretching.

Circling Ankles It's a great way to assist your ankle muscles become flexible and looser. This will also aid in increasing the circulation of blood within your lower legs as well as your feet.

1. Place your feet on the ground with their backs facing them. Stretch your right leg towards the front and bring your left knee towards your chest.

2. Inhale deeply and exhale. As you breathe out let your right ankle to turn around clockwise for 4 reps, or, if you're feeling confident eight reps.